THE INTERNATIONAL ACADEMY OF CYTOLOGY ··· 1957 ···

Acta Cytologica

The Journal of Clinical Cytology and Cytopathology

Founded 1957 by George L. Wied
Continued 2004–2013 by Marluce Bibbo

(Continued on next page)

Karger

Printed in Germany on acid-free and non-aging paper (ISO 9706) by Printec Offset, medienhaus, Kassel

Karger

www.karger.com
karger@karger.com

Acta Cytologica

National and Regional Societies and Editors

Karger

www.karger.com
karger@karger.com

Acta Cytologica

Journal Information

Aims and Scope

With articles offering an excellent balance between clinical cytology and cytopathology, *Acta Cytologica* fosters the understanding of the pathogenetic mechanisms behind cytomorphology and thus facilitates the translation of frontline research into clinical practice. As the official journal of the International Academy of Cytology and affiliated to over 50 national cytology societies around the world, *Acta Cytologica* evaluates new and existing diagnostic applications of scientific advances as well as their clinical correlations. Original papers, review articles, meta-analyses, novel insights from clinical practice, and letters to the editor cover topics from diagnostic cytopathology, gynecologic and non-gynecologic cytopathology to fine needle aspiration, molecular techniques and their diagnostic applications. As the perfect reference for practical use, *Acta Cytologica* addresses a multidisciplinary audience practicing clinical cytopathology, cell biology, oncology, interventional radiology, otorhinolaryngology, gastroenterology, urology, pulmonology and preventive medicine.

Guidelines for Authors

We strongly encourage authors to read the Guidelines for Authors at www.karger.com/acy_guidelines prior to submitting an article

Journal Contact

For questions or comments, please contact the persons responsible who can be found at http://www.karger.com/Journal/Contact/254338

ISSN Print Edition: 0001–5547
ISSN Online Edition: 1938–2650

Journal Homepage: www.karger.com/acy
Bibliographic Indices: This journal is regularly listed in bibliographic services, including Current Contents® and PubMed/MEDLINE.

Publication Data: *Acta Cytologica* is published 6 times a year. Volume 65 with 6 issues appears in 2021.

Subscription Orders:
Orders can be placed at agencies, bookstores, or directly with the Publisher.

S. Karger AG
Medical and Scientific Publishers
Allschwilerstrasse 10
CH–4009 Basel
Switzerland

t: +41 61 306 11 11
f: +41 61 306 12 34
e: karger@karger.com
w: www.karger.com

(for courier services only:
Allschwilerstrasse 10
CH–4055 Basel)

Change of Address:
Both old and new addresses should be sent to the subscription source.

Subscription Rates: Subscriptions run for a full calendar year. Prices are given per year.

Personal subscription:

Print or Online	*Print+Online combined*
CHF 493.00	CHF 567.00
EUR 452.00	EUR 520.00
USD 524.00	USD 603.00

postage and handling
(added to print and print+online)
CHF 52.80 Europe, CHF 74.40 Overseas
EUR 48.00
USD 72.00

Institutional subscription:

Print or Online	*Print+Online combined*
CHF 985.00	CHF 1133.00
EUR 904.00	EUR 1040.00
USD 1048.00	USD 1205.00

postage and handling
(added to print and print+online)
CHF 66.00 Europe, CHF 93.00 Overseas
EUR 60.00
USD 90.00

Back Volumes and Single Issues: Information on availability and prices of single print issues and print or electronic back volumes can be obtained from Customer Service at *service@karger.com*.

Karger

Acta Cytologica

Digital and Computational Cytology: What Is in the Horizon

Guest Editor
Jianyu Rao, Los Angeles, CA

31 figures, 30 in color, and 4 tables, 2021

Karger

Basel · Freiburg · Hartford · Oxford · Bangkok · Dubai · Kuala Lumpur ·
Melbourne · Mexico City · Moscow · New Delhi · Paris · Shanghai · Tokyo

S. Karger
Medical and Scientific Publishers
Basel · Freiburg · Hartford · Oxford ·
Bangkok · Dubai · Kuala Lumpur ·
Melbourne · Mexico City ·
Moscow · New Delhi · Paris ·
Shanghai · Tokyo

Disclaimer
The statements, opinions and data contained in this publication are solely those of the individual authors and contributors and not of the publisher and the editor(s). The appearance of advertisements in the journal is not a warranty, endorsement, or approval of the products or services advertised or of their effectiveness, quality or safety. The publisher and the editor(s) disclaim responsibility for any injury to persons or property resulting from any ideas, methods, instructions or products referred to in the content or advertisements.

Drug Dosage
The authors and the publisher have exerted every effort to ensure that drug selection and dosage set forth in this text are in accord with current recommendations and practice at the time of publication. However, in view of ongoing research, changes in government regulations, and the constant flow of information relating to drug therapy and drug reactions, the reader is urged to check the package insert for each drug for any change in indications and dosage and for added warnings and precautions. This is particularly important when the recommended agent is a new and/or infrequently employed drug.

Printed on acid-free and non-aging paper (ISO 9706)
ISBN 978–3–318–06673–9
e-ISBN 978–3–318–06674–6

karger@karger.com
www.karger.com/acy

Karger

Acta Cytologica

Vol. 65, No. 4, 2021

Contents

karger@karger.com
www.karger.com/acy

Karger

Cover illustration
Concept of cell classification with convolutional neural network (CNN).
Modified from Figure 2, Zhang et al., pp. 335–341.

Editorial

Acta Cytologica

Acta Cytologica 2021;65:283–285
DOI: 10.1159/000508215

Received: April 24, 2020
Accepted: April 24, 2020
Published online: July 8, 2020

Computational Technology with Artificial Intelligence and Machine Learning: What Should a Cytologist Do with It?

Jianyu Rao

Department of Pathology and Laboratory Medicine, UCLA, David Geffen School of Medicine, Los Angeles, CA, USA

There has been both hope and hype for computation, artificial intelligence (AI), and machine learning (ML) technologies in the medical field, specifically in pathology, and especially cytopathology. In 2019, the US Food and Drug Administration (FDA) released a white paper proposing a regulatory framework for AI (software) medical technologies as medical devices (software medical devices), and the report stated that AI/ML-based software medical devices will deliver safe and effective software functionality that will improve patient care [1]. For the community and academic cytologist, many questions, uncertainties, and challenges remain. What can this evolving multidisciplinary science contribute to cytology? Will this computational technology be the "third wave" or "third revolution" augmenting the first immunocytochemistry wave and the second molecular diagnostics wave? Does this technology hold a "false promise" with little, if any, practical clinical value? Alternatively, will this discipline "replace" our cytology profession and evaporate like the telephone booth as those in this technology industry often claim?

For most of us, our own life experiences serve as the foundation for our future vision. I came to the USA in early 1987 as a postdoctoral research fellow to pursue my medical career and work on fundamental cancer biomarker studies. My mentor, Dr. George P. Hemstreet III, an urologist and a pioneer in digital imaging field, developed a technique called "quantitative fluorescence image analysis (QFIA)." This system, as illustrated in Figure 1, interfaced a fluorescence microscope (Leitz) connected to a video camera, a monitor, and a computer (TAS-Plus) that was taller than myself (I am 5′7″). It was quite sophisticated at that time. The microscope was programmed automatically to scan the entire slide to capture cellular images (mainly cellular nuclei stained with Hoechst 33258), the fluorescence intensity was measured, and the image was stored in the disk (eight-inch disk, Fig. 1). The entire disk storage space was 64 kilobytes, barely enough to store 1 nuclear image, and the image analysis was "hard wired." As a comparison, a meniscus-sized iPhone chip (relative to the 8-inch disk) had a 128-gigabyte capacity. Figure 1 shows a MorphoGo system (Hangzhou, China), a combined fully automatic scanner with built-in morphology-driving cell analysis algorithms. The MorphoGo system has the capability of scanning the entire cytology slide with selected automatic single-cell acquisition, automatic optimal focusing, and automatic convolutional neural network for cellular classification. The system was originally designed to analyze bone marrow smears, including both differential count and initial diagnostic interpretation; analyze 27 slides per batch, at about 20 min per slide; and store up to 100 individual cell images per slide. More recently, the MorphoGo has been modified to analyze other less formidable sample preps, including urine, lumbar puncture fluid, and peripheral blood smears.

While the advancement of computation technologies, including computer power, the Internet, and mathematic algorithms, makes the computation cytology possible, a

karger@karger.com
www.karger.com/acy

Karger

Jianyu Rao
Department of Pathology and Laboratory Medicine, UCLA
David Geffen School of Medicine, 10833 Le Conte Ave.
Los Angeles, CA 90095 (USA)
JRao@mednet.ucla.edu

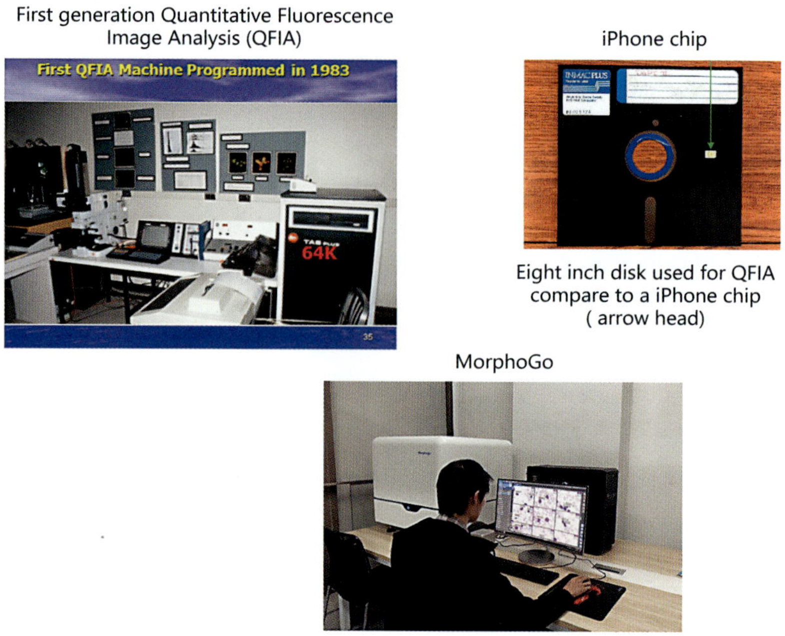

Fig. 1. Image of the QFIA system (upper left), the corresponding disk (upper right), and the MorphoGo system (bottom). QFIA, quantitative fluorescence image analysis.

technological advancement crucial for this journey is standardized sample preparation techniques, that is, liquid preparation methods. These standardized preparations produced a cell monolayer with minimum lab-to-lab variations. The combination of computation technology and the liquid-based preparation poises cytology for AI technology success, as exemplified by the cervical Pap story, elegantly reviewed by Madelyn Lew et al. in this special issue.

On the other hand, one must recognize that cellular morphology, or morphometrics, as a sole diagnostic benchmark, has its limit. Techniques that only analyze morphometrics, no matter how sophisticated the technique might be, by definition, has limitations. What I mean by that is while we can train the system to accurately distinguish cancer from non-cancer cells, it is highly unlikely that morphometrics can determine if a particular cell has HPV16 infection (not HPV18 or other type), a P53 mutation, or PDL1 overexpression purely based on morphometrics alone. In other words, in the foreseeable future, there is still a need for an educated operator (cytologist) to perform initial morphology-based examination, to determine what additional biomarkers or ancillary studies are necessary to probably perform those studies, and to integrate all the diagnostic information to guide appropriate patient management. But if the system can distinguish cancer from non-cancer cells more accurately and consistently, or give us a quantitative measurement of specific biomarker expression so that a targeted drug can be more effective, then why not?

These so-called AI technologies may be used in conjunction with other important diagnostic commodities, such as immunohistochemical or immunofluorescence staining and molecular analysis, to eventually derive the most accurate and clinically meaningful diagnosis on the cytology materials, provided the cytologists know how to apply the technology and can assemble the information together in their interpretation.

This issue reflects a first step to educate our readers and to conceptualize our creativities to optimize decisional intelligence which will mold this new science, providing high-quality validated data for economic resource utilization to develop "Digital and Computational Cytology: What Is in the Horizon"? This special edition includes a mixture of review and original research of application of AI systems for the cytological diagnosis of various organ systems. While the concept of computation and AI technologies is very broad, this treatise focuses on ML, either supervised or unsupervised, in cytological diagnosis, and areas such as ROSE or telecytology are not included. As McAlpine and Michelow [2] pointed out in their recent review: "Cytopathologists need to become informed consumers of these AI algorithms by understanding their workings and limitations, how their performance is assessed and how to validate and verify their output in clinical practice." I cannot agree more with this statement. The combination of digital morphology with quantitative biomarker analysis at the single cell level utilizing computational and AI approaches, a dream that has been relentlessly pursued by Dr. Hemstreet over 3 decades [3], may soon be realized.

Disclosure Statement

The author received travel support from Hologic Inc and Zhiwei LLC for meetings and conferences.

Author Contributions

The author prepared the entire manuscript.

References

1 Proposed regulatory framework for modifications to artificial intelligence/machine learning (AI/ML)-based software as a medical device (SaMD), discussion paper and request for feedback. US Food & Drug Administration. 2019.

2 McAlpine ED, Michelow P. The cytopathologist's role in developing and evaluating artificial intelligence in cytopathology practice. Cytopathology. 2020 Jan 19. [Epub ahead of print] Review.

3 Parry WL, Hemstreet GP 3rd. Cancer detection by quantitative fluorescence image analysis. J Urol. 1988 Feb;139(2):270–4.

Review

Acta Cytologica

Acta Cytologica 2021;65:286–300
DOI: 10.1159/000508629

Received: March 16, 2020
Accepted: May 13, 2020
Published online: July 21, 2020

Computational Cytology: Lessons Learned from Pap Test Computer-Assisted Screening

Madelyn Lew[a] David C. Wilbur[b] Liron Pantanowitz[c]

[a]Department of Pathology, University of Michigan, Ann Arbor, MI, USA; [b]Department of Pathology, Harvard Medical School, Boston, MA, USA; [c]Department of Pathology, University of Pittsburg Medical Center, Pittsburgh, PA, USA

Keywords

Artificial intelligence · Computational cytology · Computer-assisted screening · Cytology · Pap test · Screening

Abstract

Background: In the face of rapid technological advances in computational cytology including artificial intelligence (AI), optimization of its application to clinical practice would benefit from reflection on the lessons learned from the decades-long journey in the development of computer-assisted Pap test screening. ***Summary:*** The initial driving force for automated screening in cytology was the overwhelming number of Pap tests requiring manual screening, leading to workflow backlogs and incorrect diagnoses. Several companies invested resources to address these concerns utilizing different specimen processing techniques and imaging systems. However, not all companies were commercially prosperous. Successful implementation of this new technology required viable use cases, improved clinical outcomes, and an acceptable means of integration into the daily workflow of cytopathology laboratories. Several factors including supply and demand, Food and Drug Administration (FDA) oversight, reimbursement, overcoming learning curves and workflow changes associated with the adoption of new technology, and cytologist apprehension, played a significant role in either promoting or preventing the widespread adoption of automated screening technologies. ***Key Messages:*** Any change in health care, particularly those involving new technology that impacts clinical workflow, is bound to have its successes and failures. However, perseverance through learning curves, optimizing workflow processes, improvements in diagnostic accuracy, and regulatory and financial approval can facilitate widespread adoption of these technologies. Given their history with successfully implementing automated Pap test screening, cytologists are uniquely positioned to not only help with the development of AI technology for other areas of pathology, but also to guide how they are utilized, regulated, and managed.

Introduction

Pap tests were first suggested as a method of screening cervical cancer in 1928, but the test did not gain popularity until the 1940s. Since then, millions of Pap tests have been performed annually, with at least 22.6 million per-

karger@karger.com
www.karger.com/acy

Karger

Madelyn Lew
Department of Pathology, University of Michigan Health System
NCRC Bldg 35, 2800 Plymouth Road
Ann Arbor 48109 (USA)
lewm@med.umich.edu

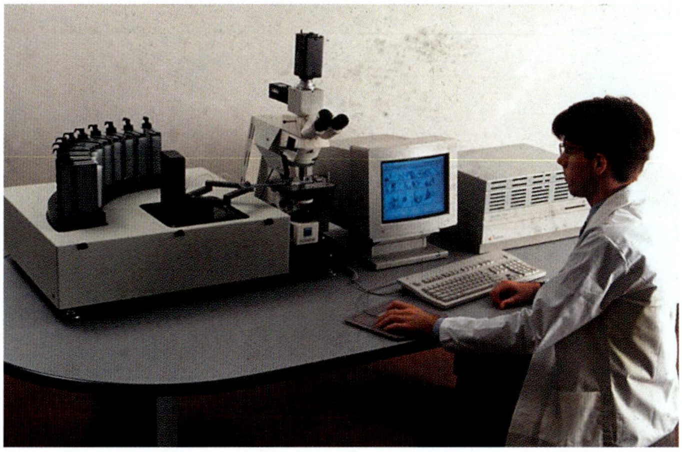

Fig. 1. A cytotechnologist shown using the first Cytyc (eventually Hologic) imaging device, a predecessor of the ThinPrep Imaging System (Imager) that never went into production. The hardware foundation of the imaging device was an Apple computer with a robotic loading arm. We thank Hologic for their permission to use this photo.

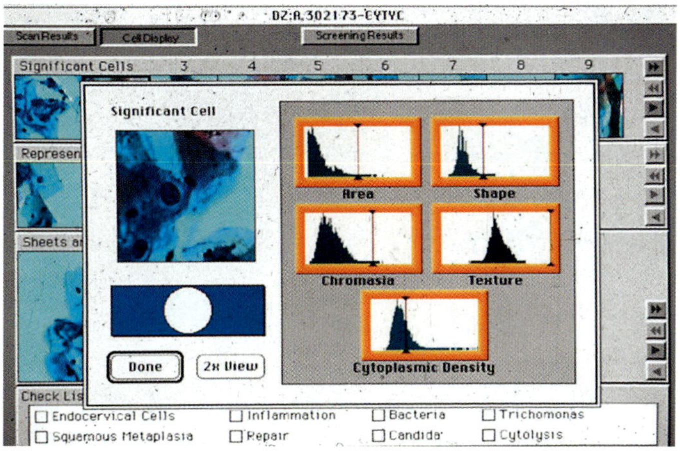

Fig. 2. Morphologic histograms resulting from the analysis of the first Cytyc (eventually Hologic) imaging device. These histograms highlight cells that have nuclear size or optical density outside of the bell curve of normal cells and flag them for review. Note that the location of these cells on the ThinPrep slide is provided. We thank Hologic for their permission to use this photo.

formed in 2016 in the USA [1]. Several decades ago, the time demand and concern regarding false-negative results in manual evaluation of Pap test specimens led to numerous investigations of alternative methods for screening cervical specimens that would enhance workflow efficiency without compromising diagnostic accuracy. Optimal screening methods needed to enhance diagnostic accuracy and reproducibility, while also facilitating cytotechnologist adherence to the newly enacted Clinical Laboratory Improvement Amendments of 1988 (CLIA88) workload legislation. The CLIA88 regulations were established to combat the hazards of work fatigue associated with long hours of screening slides, which had been shown to lead to an increase in false-negative cases. Furthermore, as the work environments of high-volume laboratories became increasingly complex and all individuals were tasked with multiple roles and responsibilities, the possibility for distractions became a bigger threat when screening Pap test slides. It is with this background pressure that automated Pap test screening became a focal point of investigation.

Today, we are embracing the era of artificial intelligence (AI) in pathology. This includes computational cytology, which combines next generation AI with digital whole slide imaging cytology. Similar applications have also been utilized in surgical pathology. Whole slide scanners can now digitize entire glass slides, creating large datasets of digitized slides that can be curated and used to better train algorithms, as well as deep learning AI models using advanced computer technology. As a result, there is great interest in applying AI tools in many areas of daily pathology practice. However, there are several formidable barriers that will need to be overcome to achieve widespread adoption. These include standardization of pre-imaging collection and preparation factors, regulatory approval, integration into routine workflow, demonstration of favorable outcomes and added value after deployment, and reimbursement that helps justify the expense of implementation. Many of these hurdles were addressed and overcome more than 2 decades ago with computer-assisted Pap test screening. Indeed, the history of automated Pap test screening has provided many lessons from which we can learn since the first commercially available automated screening systems were introduced in the 1990s.

This paper reviews the key developmental milestones of computer-assisted screening in Pap tests and highlights the important lessons learned related to Food and Drug Administration (FDA) approval, standardization of processing specimens to be imaged, overcoming workflow disruption, outcomes data following implementation, and reimbursement issues that we can apply today as we discover how best to utilize AI in other areas of pathology.

The Journey of Automated Pap Tests

First- and second-generation "image analysis" systems laid the groundwork for the first commercially available

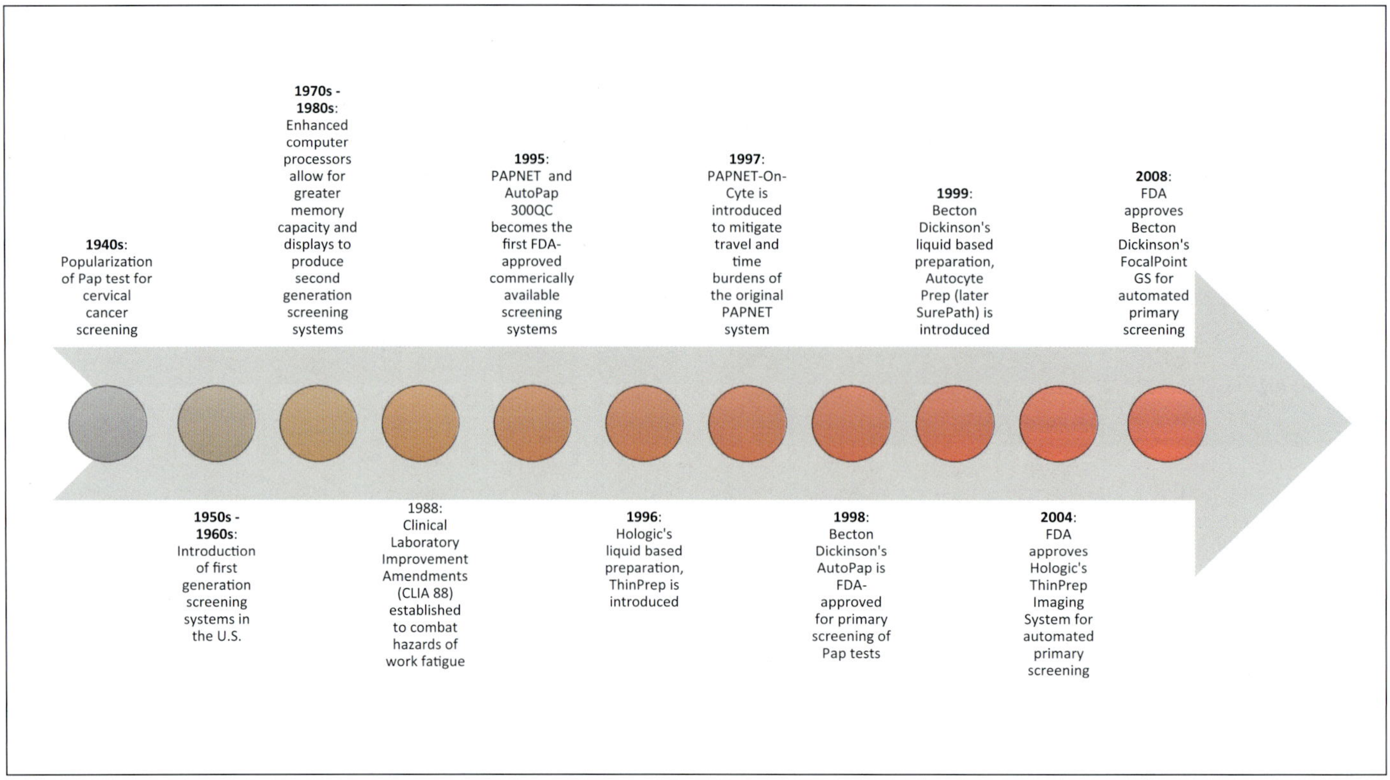

Fig. 3. Timeline of major milestones in the technologic development of automated screening of Pap tests in the United States.

automated screening system, PAPNET, that was approved for commercial use in 1992. First-generation systems included a variety of static image analyzers such as the Cytoanalyzer [2, 3], the TICAS device [4], Cell Analysis System (CAS) [5], as well as flow cytometry devices such as the slit-scan instrument [6], which were all conceived on the premise that cancer cells could be differentiated from normal cells by morphometric features such as nuclear size and optical density (Fig. 1, 2). These systems generally utilized hard-wired analogue video processing circuits and fully automated microscopes, and, in the case of slit scanning, a laminar flow tube in which cells passing through could be rapidly imaged. Each produced 2-dimensional histograms showing morphometric differences between normal and abnormal populations. Unfortunately, such systems were expensive and slow, and each produced results which were not always accurate because of the morphometric overlap between normal and neoplastic cells. Since these systems were initially conceived to produce results without human intervention, there was intense debate about whether such devices could be used clinically when these issues of inaccurate morphologic evaluation existed [7]. Inaccurate results were also attributable to the use of conventional cytology specimens as layering of cells upon one another and clustering of non-cellular materials adversely affected evaluation of cellular morphometry.

By the 1980s, computers had significantly advanced in terms of processing power and speed, memory cost and accessibility, as well as image capture and display technology. Image analytic science had dramatically progressed on other fronts, most notably in satellite reconnaissance image analysis. Two companies simultaneously developed Pap test screening systems that were directly based on such technological advances. Neuromedical Systems developed PAPNET and NeoPath developed the AutoPap (later called FocalPoint). These systems had unique approaches to evaluating a Pap test. PAPNET used neural network technology, training the system with large sets of cases of known diagnosis. Using this method, PAPNET identified individual cells of interest for display and diagnosis by cytologists. Interestingly, displays were digital, showing fields of view containing potential abnormal cells [8]. This fact made PAPNET the first truly digital pathology device. AutoPap was a device which used classifiers trained on individual cell annotations to develop algorithms from which a score of potential overall slide and individual field of view (FOV) abnormality would be determined. The algorithm was trained to give higher scores to more severe cellular abnormalities, and the higher the cumulative slide score, the more likely it was that abnormality was present somewhere on the slide. This scoring could also be extended to identify the highest scoring microscopic fields of view, which would later be used as the basis for location-guided screening applications [9]. In parallel to these computer-based technological advances, efforts were also underway to develop a better specimen for computer analysis. A group in the Netherlands introduced a new preparation method, which would later evolve into the ThinPrep Pap Test (Hologic, then Cytyc) [10, 11]. This advancement solved much of the difficulty that computers experienced with conventional smears as described above, by creating a uniform spread of cells, allowing for improved visualization of individual cell morphometry.

All of these new technologies would require substantial FDA regulatory oversight before entering the marketplace. Both PAPNET and AutoPap were conceived as and capable of primary screening in their initial configurations, but FDA needed data to evaluate the utility of these new technologies and cytologists were not adequately prepared to use such new and unvalidated methods in clinical laboratories. As such, the FDA outlined stepwise approvals beginning with "least-risk," followed by "higher-risk" use cases. Therefore, trials for both PAPNET and AutoPap were initially focused on quality control (QC) applications and led to successful approval of both devices for rescreening of conventional Pap smear preparations, which had been previously manually screened as negative as a way to reduce false-negative rates (PAPNET 1995, AutoPap 1995). Trials showed that both systems were effective in this purpose [12–15].

Unfortunately, the PAPNET system suffered from a major technological deficiency. Slides needed to be sent to a central facility for screening, after which a digital tape was returned to the participating laboratory, allowing the results to be digitally reviewed locally. This process led to suboptimal turnaround times. The QC rescreening system was also associated with high costs, estimated at USD 40,000 per life-year saved, making for very difficult laboratory implementation [13]. In 1997, there was an attempt to address the travel burden of slides by introducing the PAPNET-on-Cyte, which allowed for installation of the system in local laboratories. However, this attempt failed, as subsequent studies [14–16] supported the conclusion that the slight increase in sensitivity of detection of squamous lesions by PAPNET did not provide enough value for its overall costs. After bankruptcy in 1999, the intellectual property, patents, and assets of Neuromedical Systems were purchased by AutoCyte. This company eventually merged with NeoPath to become TriPath Imaging, which ultimately was acquired by Becton Dickinson (BD).

NeoPath initially targeted a QC application for its first commercial product, the AutoPap 300QC. This device, via its classifier algorithms, developed an overall "slide risk" score, which was proportional to the risk of that slide containing abnormal cells. The highest ranking slides initially called negative on manual review were sent for a second manual review [17]. This process was FDA approved in 1995 and had modest success in the marketplace. The subsequent FocalPoint Slide Profiler was further developed to prescreen slides, generate slide scores, and stratify the entire slide population into 3 broad categories. The lowest scoring 25% could be signed out as negative with no manual screening at all, the middle scoring population was sent for manual screening, and the highest scoring 15% were manually screened and if found to be negative, rescreened for QC purposes. Under this system, primary screening became more cost-effective as up to 25% of slides required no manual screening. However, despite the overall reliability with which the FocalPoint Slide Profiler identified low-risk slides [18], cytologists' discomfort with the lack of human review in a subset of Pap tests deterred widespread adoption of the system, leading to subsequent industrial developments in location-guided and FOV screening, which is the form cytology automation takes today.

Simultaneous to these screening technology systems, commercial development of liquid-based technology (LBC) was moving forward. While the major goal of LBC was to optimize cytology specimens for automated screening devices, clinical trials showed that LBC also provided improvement for manual screening [19]. After trials showing these results, the FDA approved ThinPrep for manual screening in 1996 and a competing product from TriPath Imaging (ultimately BD) called AutoCyte Prep (ultimately SurePath) in 1999 [20]. The first commercial products for automated primary screening using location guidance and FOV screening used these 2 products as their main specimen types – the Thin Prep Imaging System (FDA approved in 2004) and the FocalPoint GS (FDA approved in 2008) [21, 22].

The AutoPap/FocalPoint System had the ability to identify important FOVs through the use of printed

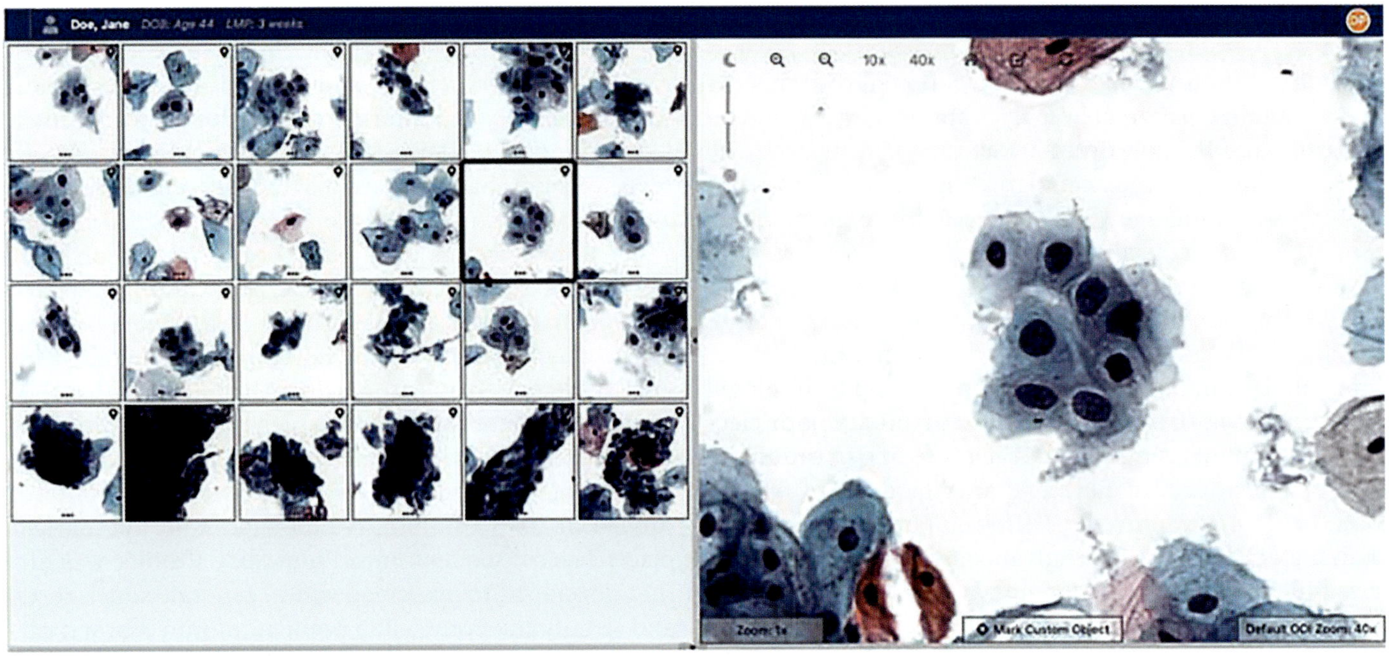

Fig. 4. Image gallery of a Pap test with HSIL shown from the developing Hologic Digital Cytology platform. The left panel shows 24 selected thumbnails including lesional cells (rows 1-3) and endocervical cells (row 4). The right whole slide image permits the cytologist access to freely navigate the entire ThinPrep cell spot.

"PAPMAPs," in which the 10 FOVs most likely to have an abnormality and 1 FOV with glandular cells could be transferred to the slide by tracing. In the commercial version of the FocalPoint GS, these were digitally transferred to a motorized stage microscope, allowing for "push-button" navigation for hierarchical review of the highest to lowest scoring FOVs. If the cytotechnologist deemed any of these predesignated areas to be abnormal, the entire slide would subsequently be manually screened. Subsequent studies touted the impact that implementation of the BD FocalPoint GS Imaging System had with improved Pap test result turnaround times, increased cytotechnologist productivity, as well as decreased false-negative rates [22, 23].

The most successful commercial application of the automated screening system, which became widely implemented in high-volume laboratories, was the Hologic (initially Cytyc) ThinPrep Imaging System (TIS), known as the Imager. Learning from the mistakes of the prior PAPNET system, TIS was installed within the local laboratory space to prevent issues with increased turnaround time attributed to slide travel. The Imager is a fundamentally different technology from the FocalPoint system, utilizing sophisticated image analysis morphometry to identify nuclear size and optical density. TIS identifies and presents, via a motorized microscope stage, 22 FOVs containing the most concerning cells identified on the slide. If the cytotechnologist deems these 22 FOVs to be normal, the slide is signed out as negative, and if there are any abnormalities, a full manual review of the slide is performed. Subsequent studies comparing the performance of the Imager with manual review generally supported the conclusion that the system enhances screening sensitivity in the detection of squamous lesions [24–27] with higher diagnostic rates of abnormal Pap tests (defined as atypical squamous cells of undetermined significance [ASC-US] or greater) [26–28].

In distinction to initial efforts, both guided screening products have been commercial successes because they enhanced cost and workflow efficiencies and increased (or at a minimum equaled) the accuracy of manual screening. As a result, the majority of Pap tests performed in the USA and many parts of the developed world now use automated guided screening with these 2 instruments, especially in commercial laboratory settings.

The review of the history of automated screening (Fig. 3) in gynecological cytology highlights how new, disruptive procedures introduced in the clinical setting require adequate time and evaluation to not only develop the technology but also identify clinically viable uses, and to allow appropriate regulatory oversight and reimbursement to be achieved. This summary will serve as background for lessons to be learned from this process in the current wave of interest and development in AI applications to pathology beyond the Pap test.

A new generation image analysis system for automated Pap test screening known as BestCyte (CellSolutions) is in development. This imaging system is comprised of a whole slide imaging scanner, networked storage, and whole slide image analysis algorithm. Abnormal cells are grouped and displayed in gallery format for end user review, which can be performed remotely using a web-based software. The software also facilitates annotation or electronic marking of cells to facilitate communication regarding cells of concern between cytotechnologists and pathologists. Additionally, the system allows for review of the entire digital slide by the cytotechnologist or pathologist [29]. CellSolutions also offers a proprietary liquid-based sample preservative solution and thin-layer slide preparation method called Glucyte, which has shown to perform reasonably well when compared to ThinPrep and SurePath slides [30, 31]. Another digital system currently under development is Hologic's Digital Cytology system for computer-assisted diagnosis of Pap tests. Hologic's new system includes a whole slide imaging scanner devoted to scanning cytologic preparations with multiple *Z* planes, which allows for superior image quality in the evaluation of 3-dimensional groups frequently found in cytologic preparations. *Z*-stacking allows acquisition of images in multiple planes, which facilitates morphologic evaluation of dense cellular aggregates (e.g., hyperchromatic crowded groups). Hologic has improved upon its currently used image analysis algorithm to analyze ThinPrep Pap test slides, the output of which no longer directs end users to use a microscope to examine specific FOVs but allows them to view images on a computer display (Fig. 4). In this system, cytologists will examine approximately 24 image tiles (snapshots) of cells instead of screening thousands of cells. If necessary, the cytologist is still able to review the entire imaged slide of the ThinPrep cell spot. While *Z*-stacking creates larger image file sizes, the enhanced image quality likely enhances the effectiveness of the image analysis algorithm. With these newer technological (e.g., *Z*-stacked image acquisition) and algorithmic (e.g., deep learning) developments, this system has the potential to enhance workflow, as it untethers the cytopathologist from a glass slide and microscope and also opens the possibility for evaluation of non-gynecological cytology cases (e.g., urine cytology and effusions) in the future with AI-based deep learning algorithms [29].

Industry Perspective

Given the current hype and funding related to AI, there are now several startup companies dedicated to developing AI tools specifically for pathology. There has also been a shift in the market because several of the long-standing digital pathology vendors have started to focus less on hardware and more on software to support computational pathology. Automation of Pap test screening is possible today because of the groundbreaking work of industry colleagues and successful academic-industry partnerships. Therefore, it is worthwhile to analyze the journeys of these companies to see if there are learned lessons that can be extrapolated to the current AI market.

Advances in digital imaging, optics, and computer technology allowed for tremendous growth in companies that were focused on digital image analysis for the evaluation of cytologic specimens. However, companies first to market learned that technological advancement alone does not ensure commercial success. As the paths of Neuromedical Systems and NeoPath illustrate, providing a rescreening system that merely increases the sensitivity for the detection of squamous lesions in Pap tests is not enough to be widely adopted. Besides providing an increased benefit in sensitivity of detecting disease processes, the system must also be easily accessible, efficient to utilize, and provide cost-benefit to health systems, which requires navigating through complex regulatory mechanisms. Both PAPNET and AutoPap technologies could have been presented as "end product" primary screening tools (as are used today) in their initial iterations. However, the FDA required a risk mitigation approach to approval, requiring additional modifications within each system to achieve their final goals. In the case of PAPNET, this required changes in product delivery. Meanwhile, changes in how slide scoring was used in the final AutoPap product went through several variations before settling on a finalized regulatory agency and consumer-acceptable version. Overall, the stepwise approval process allowed for modifications that ultimately made a more effective system as an end product.

Another important consideration for companies hoping to break into the market is the presence of existing competitors and their market penetrance. For example, the MonoPrep Pap test liquid-based preparation device (MonoGen) was approved by the FDA in 2006 [32]. Unfortunately, by this time, both ThinPrep and SurePath LBC had been in the marketplace for several years and were well accepted. For a laboratory to switch to a new preparation at this point, significant cost reduction and/

or workflow or quality advantages would be necessary. However, neither were achieved. The MonoPrep Pap test, facing this challenge, did not survive. First to market with similar devices is therefore a strong predictor of success that new AI technology will have to consider.

The TIS and FocalPoint GS (the final iteration of the AutoPap system) were both systems that survived the failures of previous screening systems. The Imager entered the regulatory process at a time when primary screening devices were well understood by the FDA, facilitating immediate offering of a product of this type. Several studies highlighted the consistency with which both systems increased screening sensitivity in detecting squamous lesions in Pap tests. Additionally, these systems were placed in local laboratories to decrease the time burdens associated with shipment of slides. The FOV-oriented guided screening approach by both vendors facilitated more efficient workflow and market acceptability by consumers [33]. For example, the TIS requires review of 22 FOVs, which accounts for approximately 25% of the evaluable slide surface area [34]. For negative Pap tests, this results in decreased screening time and enhances productivity of cytotechnologist workflow [21, 35, 36], yielding a favorable cost-to-benefit ratio when utilizing FOV-oriented screening systems. The ability of the cytologist to review morphology made for improved consumer acceptance as compared to the second-generation AutoPap Slide Profiler, which had a subset of slides that did not undergo any manual review. Several AI tools under development today are similarly focused on end user engagement and making the results of deep learning algorithms explainable to them. For example, presenting findings in the form of galleries of thumbnail images or as heat maps overlying pathology images instead of complicated histograms will likely lead to enhanced acceptance [37].

Although automated cytology companies showed that computerized screening systems could be beneficial in gynecological cytology, there is a concern today regarding the generalizability of newer AI algorithms in other areas of pathology that may not work as well when deployed in different laboratories around the world. Different specimen collection, slide preparation, and imaging processes will likely require extensive training to account for the differences in interlaboratory specimen appearances. Studies reported on most deep learning algorithms consist of models that have been trained on relatively small datasets with little heterogeneity and have been tested in limited clinical settings. As a result, these models may not be generalizable to the larger population of laboratories. Suboptimal results might be found in this setting of variable tissue preparation (e.g., section thickness and different staining) or presence of artifacts (e.g., tissue folds and regions out of focus). While computer scientists have been actively working to try to solve these problems using technology (e.g., employing data augmentation to increase datasets and color deconvolution to normalize stain differences), very little attention has been focused on improving and standardizing pre-imaging factors (e.g., fixation, slide preparation, and staining) that impact downstream AI performance. As such, a key objective gleaned from the successful models of the TIS and FocalPoint GS Imaging System is that these companies took ownership of all pre-imaging steps, allowing for wide applicability in any laboratory. These steps included sample collection in proprietary fixative (ThinPrep or SurePath), utilization of slides with pre-marked cell spots and fiducial marks to guide imaging devices (ThinPrep Imager), and standardized staining processes (Imager) or calibration steps to bring disparate stains into an acceptable range, which allowed for successful scoring (FocalPoint GS). In addition to facilitating and simplifying the ensuing image analysis phase of the Pap test process, optimization of cellular material via liquid-based collection methods provided clinical synergies that further enhanced the entire cervical cancer screening process both clinically and economically. LBC was easier for clinicians to collect, produced many fewer unsatisfactory specimens, and had the significant added benefit of providing laboratories with residual cellular material for additional studies. Such material ultimately was found useful for immunocytochemical studies and molecular testing for human papillomavirus (HPV), chlamydia, and gonorrhea. The addition of such tests immediately boosted the economic viability of the overall system as each of these components had significant clinical utility, added reimbursement, and increased the cost-benefit for the overall process [38, 39]. Ultimately, company ownership of all of the steps of the Pap test process from start to finish (i.e., specimen collection, slide processing, image analysis, and ancillary testing) allowed for a high degree of standardization and solidified these companies' presence in the everyday workflow of cytology, particularly in high-volume laboratories.

Companies planning on introducing AI-based models for additional pathology specimens need to consider these lessons on how their products fit into the overall procedures inherent in the processing of the specimens on which they are focused. Consolidation of AI products with upstream inputs and downstream results will allow for more competitive and economically viable products and wider applicability.

Successful Introduction of Products

Many companies and research laboratories are developing deep learning algorithms for pathology in hopes of bringing successful products to market. Some of these algorithms are focused on the detection of rare events (e.g., screening), while others are being designed to diagnose, grade, and quantify features such as cancer in pathology images. They promise to alleviate pathologists of mundane tasks (e.g., counting mitotic figures), eliminate negative cases to expedite workflow, or improve diagnostic accuracy and reproducibility. There are also algorithms being developed to help with prognostication directly from digital images, which is something pathologists cannot easily do today with just their light microscopes [40]. However, deep learning algorithms are frequently developed to address uses, which may be interesting from a technical or developmental aspect, but for which there is little need in routine practice. These companies and researchers therefore struggle to find appropriate purposes that would provide commercial success. Computer-assisted screening of Pap tests is a great example of where a technological solution suitably addressed a pre-existing problem, providing a perfect use case for commercial viability. The initial driving force for automated screening in cytology was the overwhelming number of Pap tests requiring manual screening by cytotechnologists, which led to workflow backlogs. Such backlogs created quality assurance issues as cytologists felt increasing time pressure to maintain acceptable turnaround times while maintaining diagnostic accuracy. Automated screening was proposed by industry to help address these work and quality demands. On one level, the widespread acceptance of LBC created slides that were generally easier to evaluate and primed cytology samples for automated screening. Meanwhile, as several studies reported, automated FOV-oriented screening of Pap tests resulted in increased workflow productivity by decreasing screening time and enhancing diagnostic accuracy. Ultimately, this led to the successful incorporation of these technologies into the daily workflow of cytology laboratories.

Learning from this lesson, companies aiming to enter the marketplace with AI products in pathology will need to assess use cases and develop applications that will have broad acceptance. Niche applications may be useful in certain settings but will struggle to achieve financial success. That being said, in common with the automated cytology example above, the industry may need to first develop technology and methods that may not apply to common and economically viable use cases in order to further develop the technology into a viable product with widespread use. Additionally, as in the automated cytology industry, iterative regulatory hurdles, industry consolidation, and the introduction of new competitors may also contribute to stepwise modification of systems to a final end product.

The Rise of Synergistic Technologies

In parallel to the development of automated screening in cytology, HPV testing dramatically shifted the demand for automated Pap test screening in another direction and continues to do so today. As the causal relationship between HPV and cervical cancer had been readily established, the American Society for Colposcopy and Cervical Pathology (ASCCP) and the American Cancer Society (ACS) released a set of treatment guidelines in 2012 that reduced the number of Pap tests needed for women in their overall lifetime via the introduction of HPV co-testing. For women 21–29 years of age, Pap tests are recommended every 3 years. For women 30–65 years of age, co-testing with cytology and HPV testing every 5 years is the preferred method of screening (although screening using cytology alone every 3 years is also acceptable) [41]. Several studies have highlighted the significant impact HPV co-testing has had on clinical workflow in cytology laboratories and clinical management. Initially, HPV testing was used as a "reflex test" to guide clinical management decisions in patients with indeterminate (ASC-US) Pap test results. However, studies that led to the management changes recommended in the updated 2012 ASCCP/ACS guidelines showed that co-testing was more sensitive for the detection of high-grade squamous intraepithelial lesions (HSIL) [42–45] and has more reproducible results than cytology alone [46, 47]. Some studies have noted that clinical triage of low-grade squamous intraepithelial lesions by HPV testing can be more sensitive for the detection of precancerous cervical lesions on subsequent biopsy than repeat cytology [48]. HPV testing's overall high sensitivity for the detection of squamous abnormalities as well as its relatively high negative predictive value has catapulted it to the frontline of screening, with some studies suggesting that it could be utilized as the main method for primary screening of cervical cancer, with cytology being more useful in identifying progressive HPV changes [49]. Such arguments are bolstered by the standardization of molecular assays for HPV in comparison to the relatively subjective visual evaluation of Pap cytology, which ultimately has led to increasing institutional and practitioner reliance on HPV testing. These practice changes have significantly reduced the number of Pap tests performed and suggest that the number of Pap tests may be further reduced by future iterations of clinical management guidelines, particularly in the HPV-vaccinated population [50]. However, it is important to note that up to 9% of patients with a negative HPV test can still have subsequent HSIL on biopsy [51]. As such, morphologic evaluation is still an important component of ensuring optimal patient care. Therefore, there still may be a demand for improved AI-based products that more reliably detect clinically significant lesions.

Although AI-based screening systems and HPV co-testing may initially be presented as competing products, the combination of these different approaches may serve to ultimately provide an effective solution. For instance, recent reports suggest that combining the results of automated screening with HPV testing may provide further workflow and accuracy improvements. In a feasibility study, the use of FocalPoint slide score added to HPV typing data has been shown to provide an equivalent "triage to colposcopy" capability as manual screening of the Pap test. Use of these 2 data points has the potential, therefore, to eliminate the manual screening process [52]. There have also been studies to support combinations of other types of tests including combining pathology with radiology data in AI-based approaches [53]. AI companies would do well to assess for such synergistic uses of different technologies, as they have the potential to improve the chances for a stronger clinical impact of their products.

Assessments of Workflow

AI-based approaches are being promoted for their potential to mitigate increased work demand attributed to a predicted pathologist shortage, growing volume of cases requiring complex ancillary testing, and the need for information required for optimal precision medicine and immuno-oncology. One of the challenges facing adoption of AI is the identification of efficient ways to integrate these tools into clinical laboratories. It is still uncertain as to whether algorithms should analyze digital images before they are seen by a human (e.g., screen slides, triage cases, and preorder stains), run only after a pathologist has seen an image and triggers a desired task (e.g., count mitoses and grade cancer), be continuously running in the background (e.g., perform ongoing cytology-histology correlations), or combinations of all the above. Some insights may be provided by looking back at how cytology laboratories integrated computer-assisted Pap test and molecular screening technologies into their practices.

Initially, manual screening of a Pap test with hierarchical review by the pathologist was the only workflow in the cytology laboratory. Initial automation devices were added as post-screen processes for QC. Evolution to a replacement for manual screening ("no review" in the FocalPoint Slide Profiler) or partial guided screening (Imager or FocalPoint GS) took place when the technology, regulatory oversight, and clinical utility were well-established. Introduction of AI-based applications in other areas of pathology will almost certainly follow this approach. Some applications may start in a QC (or "results checking") capacity and subsequently evolve into prescreening roles. Other applications will require definitive needs that can only be determined by human intervention. Examples might include ordering of a special stain or feature quantitation following the development of a differential diagnosis, analogous to ordering a HPV test in follow-up of an equivocal (ASC-US) Pap test human interpretation. Other applications might be able to predict when such tests are needed and order them following an initial prescreen without human intervention. Workflow assessment and development will be an important consideration when developers of commercial AI applications consider how to position their products in the marketplace and present them to regulators.

Workflow changes will also be implemented as AI capabilities continue to advance. Currently, automated guided screening of Pap tests is run in series with manual screening. However, commercially available systems have higher overall operational costs than manual screening alone. In a time where HPV testing and vaccination may drastically decrease the need for automated screening in its current form, different workflows that integrate AI may need to be considered in order to justify its cost in clinical settings. Since the introduction of screening systems now in commercial use, both computer power available per dollar, and AI software capabilities have increased exponentially and have led to new generation image analysis systems, which can potentially change workflow (e.g., permit cytologists to work remotely), as noted above. Another example is seen in recent publications that describe a new automated screening system for Pap tests known as the CytoProcessor™ (DATEXIM, Caen, France), which presents every individual abnormal cell detected in a gallery format ordered by severity from most concerning for high-grade to low-grade squamous lesions. If no abnormal cells are identified by the automated screening algorithm, the gallery will show no images and can thus be considered negative. In initial publications, this screening system has shown improvements in diagnostic sensitivity without changing specificity in the evaluation of Pap tests when compared to the TIS [54, 55].

Another consideration regarding the impact of technology on workflow is the potential to change the physical form the evaluated cytology specimen takes. Both the BD FocalPoint GS Imaging System and TIS were designed to evaluate glass slides. However, as rapid slide scanners allow for the opportunity to fully digitize workflow, development of newer imaging systems may completely alter workflow in laboratories and decrease slide handling tasks, further enhancing productivity and efficiency (e.g., directly analyze liquid-based cells in vials without making slides, akin to flow cytometry). Also, additional computing and scanning capacity will allow greater throughput, which can further enhance cost-benefit ratios. A digitized workflow opens up opportunities for remote evaluation with prescreened slides coupled with AI interpretations. In addition, the same digital platform used to automate Pap tests could be leveraged to run additional AI algorithms for non-gynecological samples (e.g., urine and body fluids). AI algorithms may also help augment quality assurance tasks (e.g., CLIA88-mandated 5-year look back reviews) that are currently time-consuming and tedious to perform.

Changes in Practice Associated with New Technology Introduction

With extremely limited clinical experience in using AI in anatomical pathology practice today, it is unknown whether these AI-based products will truly deliver on their promise (e.g., augmented efficiency and accuracy), or if these tools will be too disruptive to be accepted and therefore not widely implemented. Indeed, the implementation of automated Pap test screening and new specimen processing techniques introduced several changes in the daily work of cytology laboratories. One of the most notable changes was the transition from conventional smear preparations of Pap tests to LBC. This transition required an adjustment in how cytologists evaluated and interpreted morphologic features in Pap tests. While squamous abnormalities identified in ASC-US or low-grade squamous intraepithelial lesion cases are similar in conventional smear preparations and LBC, significant differences have been noted in cases of HSIL and squamous cell carcinoma. Fewer numbers of HSIL cells were present in LBC, which often occurred singly or in small cell groups in LBC, leading to either misclassification as benign glandular cells or macrophages or being overlooked entirely on manual screening [56]. Other studies noted additional cytomorphologic differences in HSIL cells in LBC compared to conventional smear preparations (e.g., darker staining, smaller nuclear areas, less distinct nuclear chromatin, and thicker 3-dimensional groupings in LBC), which may make detection of these lesional cells more difficult [57, 58]. While these changes in morphologic evaluation could have hindered the use of LBC in gynecological cytology, the significant benefits imparted by its adoption such as decreased number of unsatisfactory specimens, enhanced visualization of cells, and increased productivity [59], in conjunction with the ability to utilize residual specimen for ancillary testing, justified the adjustment of diagnostic criteria. After appropriate training of cytologists, studies have shown a higher rate of detection for squamous abnormalities in LBC compared to conventional smear preparations [19, 60–62]. This experience highlights how integration of new technology can actually impact diagnostic criteria and, more importantly, how a positive approach to working through learning curves associated with new technology and workflows can benefit health-care delivery in the long run.

AI-based applications may also cause shifts in fundamental ways specimens are examined. One example that has emerged is in the area of breast cancer interpretation. In a study of unsupervised AI evaluation of breast cancers with known outcomes, computational pathology algorithms pointed out that stromal changes were found to be more predictive of those outcomes than standardly used methods such as tumor grading, giving rise to a previously unrecognized prognostic determinant and potentially shifting morphologic criteria for evaluation [40]. It is likely that many other findings such as these will force changes in the underlying knowledge and practice patterns that will emerge from a new way of looking at digitized images.

Regulations and Reimbursement

The FDA approval processes for extant automated screening devices detailed above will likely mirror the approval path that will be applied to AI-based technology. We have already seen approvals of the first devices for the

Acta Cytologica 2021;65:286–300
DOI: 10.1159/000508629

primary interpretation of whole slide images [63, 64]. The first application required a non-inferiority clinical trial in support of a premarket approval, which is the most stringent level of FDA clearance. Already, the expectations and requirements have been lowered with subsequent applications, which have required the less intense 510k level of approval. AI-based software applications will most likely follow a similar course. As the FDA becomes more expert in evaluating new AI-based digital pathology applications for use, the paths to approval will hopefully become clearer, offering companies a better understanding of the bars to be hurdled. Of course, individual laboratories may develop their own AI-based applications as laboratory developed tests for internal use. However, if broad applicability and commercialization is the desired route, FDA oversight will be necessary. Currently, it is unclear if the FDA process will tether AI applications to specific imaging devices and permit adaptive algorithms that can continually learn and improve over time. Such decisions may impact the speed and extent of incorporating AI into pathology in the future.

Regulatory oversight of laboratory operations (the purview of CLIA88) also has important implications learned from cytology automation. For instance, if an AI-based product were to be developed for prescreening digital prostate core biopsies and showing areas of high probability for cancer (the exact correlate of guided screening in cytology), the pathologist should be able to review more prostate biopsies. But how many would be safe? At present, there are no regulations regarding pathologist workload. Such regulation could be added as methods change, particularly with the potential for misuse of a prescreening technology. This scenario has already been addressed in the story of automated cytology. As described above, the drive for cytology automated screening came from the increasing workload demands on cytotechnologists. To address this, companies producing automated screening technology highlighted the substantial increase in productivity as one of its major advantages. Noting that automated screening decreased cytotechnologist screening time for negative Pap tests, in 2010, the Centers for Medicare and Medicaid Services (CMS) made adjustments to the original screening limitations put forth in CLIA88. These new regulations counted each negative Pap test evaluated by automated screening as half a slide, whereas each slide that underwent subsequent full manual review would be counted as one and half slides to account for efforts attributed to both automated and manual screening. While these numbers were initially presented as protective limits for cytotechnologists, some laboratories began using them as productivity targets. This led to an increased number of false negatives as fewer Pap tests underwent full manual review [65, 66]. As a result, recommendations for cytotechnologists' automated screening workloads were introduced by the American Society of Cytopathology (ASC) to ensure safe performance expectations. These recommendations stated that average cytotechnologist productivity should not exceed 70 slides per day when calculated using the modified workload regulations defined by the CMS 2010 adjustments, and that the percentage of slides undergoing full manual review should be either >15% or twice the percentage of cases interpreted as cytologically abnormal. Interestingly, laboratories adhering to these recommendations may not show a substantial benefit in workflow productivity when using automated screening, countering one of the initially touted benefits of the automated screening process. AI product developers should be aware of the consequences of products touting improvements in a particular area, which may ultimately lead to negative impacts in other areas.

Deploying AI technology for routine use in anatomical pathology has the potential for financial challenges, including the high costs associated with investing in information technology infrastructure and architecture (e.g., cloud computing, computer servers, and storage). It is unclear how these costs will be justified and whether a return on investment will come directly from additional reimbursement for using specific AI applications or by indirect means such as improved workflow efficiency. It is therefore worth reviewing how these financial burdens were addressed when cytology laboratories transitioned to using computer-assisted screening. When a Pap test is performed and evaluated by a laboratory, the technical service is reimbursed via the American Medical Association's Current Procedural Terminology (CPT) coding system, through which a specified allocation for reimbursement is made. The amount allocated is determined by a variety of factors, which may include the reporting system utilized, evaluation methods, and whether a rescreen is necessary. CPT codes are not just created when new technologies appear. Automated cytology companies needed to apply for the generation of these codes. Applications are made to the RVS Update Committee of the American Medical Association (AMA) ("the RUC"). As described on the AMA website, the RUC is a "unique multispecialty committee dedicated to describing the resources required to provide physician services which the Centers for Medicare & Medicaid Services (CMS) considers in developing Relative Value Units (RVUs) [67]." CPT codes previously existed and were valued for manual screening of Pap tests but had to be created (and valued) for automated review. Companies selling automated Pap test systems made presentations at the RUC meetings, detailing descriptions of the products and processes with recommended code valuations. The RUC then determined if such codes were warranted and how they should be scaled. The RUC makes recommendations, but CMS makes final determinations about levels of reimbursement in the Medicare system. Private insurers may follow Medicare or may decide differently. Therefore, companies made strong efforts in these presentations to the RUC, CMS, and to private insurers in order to (1) obtain CPT codes, (2) to value the CPT codes, (3) to obtain a value for the codes from CMS that insured financial viability of the product, and (4) to convince private insurers to also reimburse for the services. Item #4 was often tied to independent assessments made by the private insurers (e.g., Blue Cross/Blue Shield Technology Assessment Committee evaluations). This process can be a lengthy one and, in the case of automated Pap test screening, was an ongoing process which paralleled, rather than followed, development of the products. Fortunately, automated Pap test screening CPT codes were created by the above process and were ultimately valued at nearly 2 times the level of manual screening, creating a path to financial success. AI-based products seeking to be marketed commercially will undoubtedly require a similar path to reimbursement levels that will insure viability.

Practitioner Mindset

Many pathologists today have concerns about AI use in routine clinical practice. These include not knowing what is inside the "black box" of AI applications, ethics of its use, uncertainty about liability, the risk of becoming deskilled, and even the threat of being entirely replaced. In the past few years, several mainstream articles have postulated that AI will displace much of the work doctors do, particularly those in radiology and pathology. The authors of these articles state that complex algorithms can provide objective data that will exceed the diagnostic accuracy of humans in these fields [68]. Ardila et al. [69] reported that deep learning algorithms could outperform 6 trained radiologists with significant decreases in false positives and negatives when prior computed tomography images were not available for review. Other studies have lauded the diagnostic accuracy of AI in other realms of radiology and clinical practices like dermatology, yielding comparable or better results when compared to experienced clinicians [70, 71]. When computer-assisted screening of Pap tests was first introduced into cytology laboratories, there were skeptics. However, after this technology was deployed and cytology end users overcame their learning curve, these systems became entrenched in many laboratories. They were particularly helpful in high volume settings with favorable financial gains.

Some research groups have noted that algorithms and neural networks can provide objectively defined sets of data in the evaluation of histologic tissue, leading to more consistent diagnoses in multiple organ sites, including Gleason scoring of prostate cancer [72, 73]. These authors note that algorithmic evaluation of pathology specimens by computers can allow for integration of quantitative data from both morphologic and molecular datasets, as discussed above, to provide predictive personalized reports. However, they also acknowledge that the role of the pathologist as a diagnostician will not be lost in this future method of practice. Rather, these technologies will be applied as part of the pathologist diagnostic tool kit in order to augment diagnostic accuracy. The development of such tools has the potential to decrease subjectivity and diagnostic "grey zones" of disease processes by providing more quantitative data. Additionally, with the increasing amount of specimens to be evaluated by a diminishing population of pathologists globally, these tools can help enhance efficiency [74], which would be particularly beneficial in locations where there is a shortage of pathologists. Similar to the introduction of other technologies that initially induced fear of replacement, such as molecular testing and immunohistochemistry, the diagnostic potential of automated screening and AI-based pathology applications will require oversight by pathologists in order to make sure that these systems are valuable, relevant, and safe.

Conclusions

In reflecting on the developmental milestones of imaging systems dedicated to automated screening of Pap tests, there are clearly numerous valuable lessons we have learned (Table 1) that can be applied today toward understanding how best to use AI in pathology. As with any change, especially involving new technology that impacts workflows, there are bound to be both successes and failures. This applies to both industry and laboratory partners along the journey. In industry, history has shown

Table 1. Lessons learned about adopting AI from computer-assisted Pap test screening

What happened	Lesson learned
Computer-assisted Pap test screening solved the bottleneck of delayed time to manually screen cases as well as improve accuracy	It is important to design tools using newer technology that satisfy a gap or solve a real problem. Forcing end users to try use tools just because they are novel is unlikely to secure adoption and avoids falling into the trap of the "shiny object syndrome"
Despite showing initial promise, some systems such as PAPNET and MonoPrep did not succeed commercially. The high cost and high turnaround time of these early systems are some of the reasons that precluded their widespread adoption	Not all companies that produce technology products will be successful, particularly if the product is hard to use, is expensive, and disrupts workflow. First generation systems are also unlikely to be the final technology solution that is permanently adopted
Successful companies such as BD and Hologic created innovative computer-assisted Pap test screening systems that incorporated cytotechnologists into their workflow	Companies are more likely to succeed when their technology is designed to adapt to the needs and workflows of clients/laboratories
Companies producing computer-assisted Pap test screening devices also created new specimen processing pathways that facilitated imaging and analysis of cytology slides. Liquid-based cytology thereby helped standardize specimens that were easier to image due to less artifacts	Industrial ownership of all steps of a process from pre-imaging steps to digital image analysis helps guarantee success of the end product
Integration of computer-assisted Pap test screening disrupted previously established laboratory workflow	Integration of any new technology or innovative process will disrupt workflow, but this is likely to be short-lived after end users overcome an initial learning curve
Utilization of technology increased Pap test accuracy and decreased false-negative rates	If implemented well, AI has the potential to improve diagnostic accuracy and productivity in the pathology laboratory
Applying technology to routine practice boosted cytotechnologist productivity. However, misuse of increased screening limits led to false-negative cases	The cytology profession responded to increased cytotechnologist workloads by modifying workload limits. We should therefore be cautious about what we wish for when deploying AI tools
Algorithms trained to specifically detect squamous lesions sometimes missed rare glandular lesions in Pap tests, because they were not designed for this specific purpose	Most AI algorithms are designed to perform 1 key task. Such focused AI is known as weak or narrow AI. Strong AI refers to machines that can think like humans
CPT codes were introduced that allowed for reimbursement of automated screening	Without sufficient reimbursement to address the costs associated with purchasing new technologies, laboratories may be reluctant to implement these systems
The FDA approved computerized systems that employed image analysis as an aid to screen Pap tests, but did so in a staged manner, allowing the development of regulatory expertise	The willingness of the FDA to approve computer-assisted technology for diagnostic use sets a positive precedent for future regulatory approval of AI tools to be used in the laboratory. Developers must be aware that a staged approach may be necessary

how the commercial success of a given system depends not only on its technical merit but also by an appropriate use case, the ease with which it can integrate into daily workflow, and how well it is accepted by end users. Also, given the high upfront costs of investing in these systems, their results must be justifiable with appropriate cost-benefit. In the future, financial success will require generation of new CPT coding and obtaining appropriate reimbursement. For individual laboratories, the introduction of any new technology will introduce changes into daily workflow. While there will be some early growing pains as pathologists adapt to these changes, it is anticipated that, over time, AI tools will be increasingly adopted, allowing the field to capitalize on their many strengths. When it comes to embracing novel technology, the cytology community is clearly an early adopter. Cytologists are therefore uniquely positioned to not only help direct the development of AI algorithms but also to provide guidance in the process of successful implementation.

Conflict of Interest Statement

L.P. is on the medical advisory board of Ibex and consults for Hamamatsu. D.C.W. is the Chief Scientist of Corista LLC and a consultant to VisionGate.

Funding Sources

The authors did not receive any funding..

Author Contributions

M.L.: Acquisition, analysis, and interpretation of resource materials to the review article. Drafted the manuscript and contributed significant revisions on subsequent drafts. Contributed to final approval of version to be published. Agrees to be accountable for all aspects of the work in ensuring questions related to accuracy or integrity of any part of the work are appropriately investigated and resolved. D.C.W.: Acquisition, analysis, and interpretation of resource materials to the review article. Contributed critical revisions for important intellectual content. Contributed to final approval of version to be published. Agrees to be accountable for all aspects of the work in ensuring questions related to accuracy or integrity of any part of the work are appropriately investigated and resolved. L.P.: Designed conception of review article. Contributed critical revisions for important intellectual content. Contributed to final approval of version to be published. Agrees to be accountable for all aspects of the work in ensuring questions related to accuracy or integrity of any part of the work are appropriately investigated and resolved.

References

1 Centers for Disease Control and Prevention. National ambulatory medical care survey: 2016 national summary tables. [cited 2020 Jan 13]. Available from: www.cdc.gov/nchs/data/ahcd/namcs_summary/2016_namcs_web_tables.pdf.
2 Spencer CC, Bostrom RC. Performance of the cytoanalyzer in recent clinical trials. J Natl Cancer Inst. 1962;29:267–76.
3 Bengtsson E, Malm P. Screening for cervical cancer using automated analysis of PAP-smears, Comput Math Methods Med. 2014; 2014:842037.
4 Wied Gl, Bartels PH, Bahr GF, Oldfield DG. Taxonomic intra-cellular analytic system (TICAS) for cell identification. Acta Cytol. 1968; 12(3):180–204, 208–217, 393–412.
5 Bacus JW, Bacus JV. Quality control in image cytometry: DNA ploidy. J Cell Biochem Suppl. 1994;19:153–64
6 Wheeless LL Jr, Reeder JE, O'Connell MJ. Slit-scan flow analysis of cytologic specimens from the female genital tract. Methods Cell Biol. 1990;33:501–7.
7 Wilbur DC. Dr. Bibbo's presidential address on automation in cytology: were her predictions right, wrong, or somewhere in the middle? Acta Cytol. 2017;61(4–5):345–58.
8 Koss LG, Lin E, Schreiber K, Elgert P, Mango L. Evaluation of the PAPNET cytologic screening system for quality control of cervical smears. Am J Clin Pathol. 1994;101(2):220–9
9 Pattern SF Jr, Lee JS, Nelson AC. NeoPath, Inc. NeoPath AutoPap 300 automatic pap screener system. Acta Cytol.1996;40:45–52.
10 Oud PS, Zahniser DJ, Haag DJ, van Boekel MC, Hermkens HG, Herman CJ, et al. A new disaggregation device for cytology specimens. Cytometry. 1984;5(5):509–14.
11 Hutchinson ML, Isenstein LM, Goodman A, Hurley AA, Douglass KL, Mui KK, et al. Homogeneous sampling accounts for the increased diagnostic accuracy using the ThinPrep Processor. Am J Clin Pathol. 1994; 101(2):215–9.
12 Marshall CJ, Rowe L, Bentz JS. Improved quality-control detection of false-negative Pap smears using the Autopap 300 QC system. Diagn Cytopathol. 1999;20(3):170–4.
13 Mango LJ, Radensky P. Neural network-assisted ("NNA") analysis of cervical smears: pooled effectiveness results and economic analysis. Prim Care Update Ob Gyns. 1998; 5(4):162–3.
14 Troni GM, Cipparrone I, Cariaggi MP, Ciatto S, Miccinesi G, Zappa M, et al. Detection of false-negative Pap smears using the PAPNET system. Tumori. 200;86(6):455–7.
15 Mitchell H, Medley G. Detection of laboratory false negative smears by the PAPNET cytologic screening system. Acta Cytol. 1998; 42(1):65–70.
16 Brotzman GL, Kretzchmar S, Ferguson D, Gottlieb M, Stowe C. Costs and outcomes of PAPNET secondary screening technology for cervical cytologic evaluation. A community hospital's experience. Arch Fam Med. 1999;8(1):52–5.
17 Wilbur DC, Bonfiglio TA, Rutkowski MA, Atkison KM, Richart RM, Lee JS, et al. Sensitivity of the AutoPap 300 QC System for cervical cytologic abnormalities. Biopsy data confirmation. Acta Cytol. 1996;40(1):127–32.
18 Wilbur DC. Automated cervical cancer screening: apprehension or logic: which will it be? Diagn Cytopathol. 1999;21(4):235–7.
19 Wilbur DC, Cibas ES, Merritt S, James LP, Berger BM, Bonfiglio TA. ThinPrep processor. Clinical trials demonstrate an increased detection rate of abnormal cervical cytologic specimens. Am J Clin Pathol. 1994;101(2):209, 14.
20 Tench W. Preliminary assessment of the AutoCyte PREP. Direct-to-vial performance. J Reprod Med. 2000;45(11):912–6
21 Biscotti CV, Dawson AE, Dziura B, Galup L, Darragh T, Rahemtulla A, et al. Assisted primary screening using the automated ThinPrep Imaging System. Am J Clin Pathol. 2005; 123(2):281–7.
22 Wilbur DC, Black-Schaffer WS, Luff RD, Abraham KP, Kemper C, Molina JT, et al. The Becton Dickinson FocalPoint GS Imaging System: clinical trials demonstrate significantly improved sensitivity for the detection of important cervical lesions. Am J Clin Pathol. 2009;132(5):767–75.
23 Wong R, Levi AW, Harigopal M, Schofield K, Chhieng DC. The positive impact of simultaneous implementation of the BD FocalPoint GS Imaging System and lean principles on the operation of gynecologic cytology. Arch Pathol Lab Med. 2012;136(2):183–9.
24 Dziura B, Quinn S, Richard K. Performance of an imaging system vs. manual screening in the detection of squamous intraepithelial lesions of the uterine cervix. Acta Cytol. 2006; 50(3):309–11.
25 Chivukula M, Saad RS, Elishaev E, White S, Mauser N, Dabbs DJ. Introduction of the Thin Prep Imaging System (TIS): experience in a high volume academic practice. Cytojournal. 2007;4:6.
26 Duby JM, DiFurio MJ. Implementation of the ThinPrep Imaging System in a tertiary military medical center. Cancer. 2009;117(4):264–70.
27 Pacheco MC, Conley RC, Pennington DW, Bishop JW. Concordance between original screening and final diagnosis using imager vs. manual screen of cervical liquid-based cytology slides. Acta Cytol. 2008;52(5):575–8.
28 Davey E, d'Assuncao J, Irwig L, Macaskill P, Chan SF, Richards A, et al. Accuracy of reading liquid based cytology slides using the ThinPrep Imager compared with conventional cytology: prospective study. BMJ. 2007; 335(7609):31.
29 Pantanowtiz L, Bui MM. Computer-assisted pap test screening. In: Bui MM, Pantanowitz L, editors. Modern techniques in cytopathology. Monogr Clin Cytol. Basel, Switzerland: Karger; 2020. Vol. 25; p. 67–74.
30 Alaghehbandan R. Performance of the CellSolutions Glucyte liquid-based cytology in comparison with the ThinPrep and SurePath methods. Acta Cytol. 2013;57(2):189–97.
31 Delga A, Goffin F, Kridelka F, Maree R, Lambart C, Delvenne P. Evaluations of CellSolutions BestPrep automated thin-layer liquid based cytology Papanicolaou slide preparations and BestCyte cell sorter imaging system. Acta Cytol. 2015;58(5):469–77.
32 Cibas ES, Alonzo TA, Austin RM, Bolick DR, Glant MD, Henry MR, et al. The MonoPrep Pap test for the detection of cervical cancer and its precursors. Part I: results of a multicenter clinical trial. Am J Clin Pathol. 2008; 129(2):193–201.
33 Sweeney BJ, Wilbur DC. Effects on cervical cytology screening productivity associated with implementation of the BD FocalPoint™ Guided Screener Imaging System. Acta Cytol. 2013;57(2):147–52.
34 Dawson AE. Can we change the way we screen?: the ThinPrep Imaging System. Cancer. 2004;102(6):340–4.

35 Schledermann D, Hyldebrandt T, Ejersbo D, Hoelund B, Automated screening versus manual screening: a comparison of the ThinPrep imaging system and manual screening in a time study. Diagn Cytopathol. 2007;35(6):348–52.
36 Bolger N, Heffron C, Regan I, Sweeney M, Kinsella S, McKeown M, et al. Implementation and evaluation of a new automated interactive image analysis system. Acta Cytol. 2006;50(5):483–91.
37 Cengel KA, Day SJ, Davis-Devine S, Adams CL, Madison-Henness D, Hartman ME, et al. Effectiveness of the SurePath liquid-based Pap test in automated screening and in detection of HSIL. Diagn Cytopathol. 2003;29(5):250–5.
38 Limaye A, Connor AJ, Huang X, Luff R. Comparative analysis of conventional Papanicolaou tests and a fluid-based thin-layer method. Arch Pathol Lab Med. 2003;127(2):200–4.
39 Keyhani-Rofagha S, Vesey-Shecket M. Diagnostic value, feasibility, and validity of preparing cell blocks from fluid-based gynecologic cytology specimens. Cancer. 2002;96(4):204–9.
40 Beck AH, Sangoi AR, Leung S, Marinelli RJ, Nielsen TO, van de Vijver MJ, et al. Systematic analysis of breast cancer morphology uncovers stromal features associated with survival. Sci Transl Med. 2011;3(108):108ra113.
41 Saslow D, Solomon D, Lawson HW, Killackey M, Kulasingam SL, Cain J, et al. American Cancer Society, American Society for Colposcopy and Cervical Pathology, and American Society for Clinical Pathology screening guidelines for the prevention and early detection of cervical cancer. Am J Clin Pathol. 2012;137(4):516–42.
42 Cuzick J, Clavel C, Petry KU, Meijer CJ, Hoyer H, Ratnam S, et al. Overview of the European and North American studies on HPV testing in primary cervical cancer screening. Int J Cancer. 2006;119(5):1095–101.
43 Naucler P, Ryd W, Törnberg S, Strand A, Wadell G, Elfgren K, et al. Human papillomavirus and Papanicolaou tests to screen for cervical cancer. N Engl J Med. 2007;357(16):1589–97.
44 Bulkmans NW, Berkhof J, Rozendaal L, van Kemenade FJ, Boeke AJ, Bulk S, et al. Human papillomavirus DNA testing for the detection of cervical intraepithelial neoplasia grade 3 and cancer: 5-year follow-up of a randomised controlled implementation trial. Lancet. 2007;370(9601):1764–72.
45 Castle PE, Stoler MH, Wright TC Jr, Sharma A, Wright TL, Behrens CM. Performance of carcinogenic human papillomavirus (HPV) testing and HPV16 or HPV18 genotyping for cervical cancer screening of women aged 25 years and older: a subanalysis of the ATHENA study. Lancet Oncol. 2011;12(9):880–90.
46 Stoler MH. HPV for cervical cancer screening: is the era of the molecular pap smear upon us? J Histochem Cytochem. 2001;49(9):1197–8.
47 Carozzi FM, Del Mistro A, Confortini M, Sani C, Puliti D, Trevisan R, et al. Reproducibility of HPV DNA testing by hybrid capture 2 in a screening setting. Am J Clin Pathol. 2005; 124(5):716–21.
48 Kelly RS, Patnick J, Kitchener HC, Moss SM. HPV testing as a triage for borderline or mild dyskaryosis on cervical cytology: results from the Sentinel Sites study. Br J Cancer. 2011; 105(7):983–8.
49 Huh WK, Ault KA, Chelmow D, Davey DD, Goulart RA, Garcia FA, et al. Use of primary high-risk human papillomavirus testing for cervical cancer screening: interim clinical guidance. Gynecol Oncol. 2015;136(2):178–82.
50 Chrysostomou AC, Stylianou DC, Constantinidou A, Kostrikis LG. Cervical cancer screening Programs in Europe: the transition towards HPV vaccination and population-based HPV testing. Viruses. 2018;10(12):729.
51 Sun H, Masand RP, Patel SJ, Padmanabhan V. High grade squamous intraepithelial lesion on high-risk HPV negative patients: why we still need the Pap test. Diagn Cytopathol. 2018;46(11):908–13.
52 Schiffman M, Yu K, Zuna R, Terence Dunn S, Zhang H, Walker J, et al. Proof-of-principle study of a novel cervical screening and triage strategy: computer-analyzed cytology to decide which HPV-positive women are likely to have ≥CIN2. Int J Cancer. 2017;140(3):718–25.
53 Khorrami M, Prasanna P, Gupta A, Patil P, Velu PD, Thawani R, et al. Changes in CT radiomic features associated with lymphocyte distribution predict overall survival and response to immunotherapy in non-small cell lung cancer. Cancer Immunol Res. 2020;8(1): 108–19.
54 Crowell EF, Bazin C, Saunier F, Brixtel R, Caillot Y, Lesner B, et al. CytoProcessorTM: a new cervical cancer screening system for remote diagnosis. Acta Cytol. 2019;63(3):215–23.
55 Crowell EF, Bazin C, Thurotte V, Elie H, Jitaru L, Olivier G, et al. Adaptation of cytoProcessor for cervical cancer screening of challenging slides. Diagn Cyto. 2019;47:890–7.
56 Mulford DK. Alternatives to the traditional Papanicolaou (pap) smear: liquid based cytology (LBC). Lab Med. 2003;34(2):129–31.
57 Malle D, Pateinakis P, Chakka E, Destouni C. Experience with a thin-layer, liquid-based cervical cytologic screening method. Acta Cytol. 2003;47(2):129–34.
58 Wilbur DC, Dubeshter B, Angel C, Atkison KM. Use of thin-layer preparations for gynecologic smears with emphasis on the cytomorphology of high-grade intraepithelial lesions and carcinomas. Diagn Cytopathol. 1996;14(3):201–11.
59 Singh VB, Gupta N, Nijhawan R, Srinivasan R, Suri V, Rajwanshi A. Liquid-based cytology versus conventional cytology for evaluation of cervical Pap smears: experience from the first 1000 split samples. Indian J Pathol Microbiol. 2015;58(1):17–21.
60 Azlin T, Smith S, Lambird PA. A comparison study of gynecologic specimens using the Roche Cyto-Rich monolayer Papanicolaou smear and the conventional Papanicolaou smear methods. Acta Cytol. 1994;38:805.
61 Bolick DR, Hellman DJ. Laboratory implementation and efficacy assessment of the ThinPrep cervical cancer screening system. Acta Cytol. 1993;42(1):209–13.
62 Marino JF, Fremont-Smith M. Direct-to-vial experience with AutoCyte PREP in a small New England regional cytology practice. J Reprod Med. 2001;46(4):353–8.
63 Evans AJ, Bauer TW, Bui MM, Cornish TC, Duncan H, Glassy EF, et al. US food and drug administration approval of whole slide imaging for primary diagnosis: a key milestone is reached and new questions are raised. Arch Pathol Lab Med. 2018;142(11):1383–7.
64 Imaging Technology News. Leica biosystems received FDA clearance for aperio AT2 DX digital pathology system. [cited 2020 Feb 23]. Available from: https://www.itnonline.com/content/leica-biosystems-receives-fda-clearance-aperio-at2-dx-digital-pathology-system. Published May 29, 2019.
65 Elsheikh TM, Kirkpatrick JL, Cooper MK, Johnson ML, Hawkins AP, Renshaw AA. Increasing cytotechnologist workload above 100 slides per day using the ThinPrep Imaging System leads to significant reductions in screening accuracy. Cancer Cytopathol. 2010:118(2):75–82.
66 Levi AW, Galullo P, Gordy K, Mikolaiski N, Schofield K, Elsheikh TM, et al. Increasing cytotechnologist workload above 100 slides per day using the BD FocalPoint GS imaging system negatively affects screening performance. Am J Clin Pathol. 2012;138(6):811–5.
67 American Medical Association. RVUS update committee (RUC). [cited 2020 Feb 23]. Available from: https://www.ama-assn.org/about/rvs-update-committee-ruc.
68 Obermeyer Z, Emanuel EJ. Predicting the future: big data, machine learning, and clinical medicine. N Engl J Med. 2016;375(13):1216–9.
69 Ardila D, Kiraly AP, Bharadwaj S, Choi B, Reicher JJ, Peng L, et al. End-to-end lung cancer screening with three-dimensional deep learning on low-dose chest computed tomography. Nat Med. 2019;25(6):954–61.
70 Rodriguez-Ruiz A, Lång K, Gubern-Merida A, Broeders M, Gennaro G, Clauser P, et al. Stand-alone artificial intelligence for breast cancer detection in mammography: comparison with 101 radiologists. Jorn Nat Can Inst. 2019;111(9):916–22.
71 Esteva A, Kuprel B, Novoa RA, Ko J, Swetter SM, Blau HM, et al. Dermatologist-level classification of skin cancer with deep neural networks. Nature. 2017;542(7639):115–8.
72 Saidi O, Cordon-Cardo C, Costa J. Technology insight: will systems pathology replace the pathologist? Nat Clin Pract Urol. 2007;4(1): 39–45.
73 Doyle S, Feldman M, Tomaszewski J, Madabhushi A. A boosted Bayesian multiresolution classifier for prostate cancer detection from digitized needle biopsies. IEEE Trans Biomed Eng. 2012;59(5):1205–18.
74 Hipp J, Flotte T, Monaco J, Cheng J, Madabhushi A, Yagi Y, et al. Computer aided diagnostic tools aim to empower rather than replace pathologists: lessons learned from computational chess. J Pathol Inform. 2011;2:25.

Review

Acta Cytologica

Acta Cytologica 2021;65:301–309
DOI: 10.1159/000510991

Received: May 28, 2020
Accepted: August 18, 2020
Published online: November 2, 2020

Challenges Developing Deep Learning Algorithms in Cytology

Ewen David McAlpine[a] Liron Pantanowitz[b] Pamela M. Michelow[a]

[a]Division of Anatomical Pathology, School of Pathology, University of the Witwatersrand and National Health Laboratory Service, Johannesburg, South Africa; [b]Department of Pathology, University of Michigan, Ann Arbor, MI, USA

Keywords

Algorithms · Artificial intelligence · Deep learning · Digital pathology · Digital cytology

Abstract

Background: The incorporation of digital pathology into routine pathology practice is becoming more widespread. Definite advantages exist with respect to the implementation of artificial intelligence (AI) and deep learning in pathology, including cytopathology. However, there are also unique challenges in this regard. ***Summary:*** This review discusses cytology-specific challenges, including the need to implement digital cytology prior to AI; the large file sizes and increased acquisition times for whole slide images in cytology; the routine use of multiple stains, such as Papanicolaou and Romanowsky stains; the lack of high-quality annotated datasets on which to train algorithms; and the considerable computer resources required, in terms of both computer infrastructure and skilled personnel, for computing and storage of data. Global concerns regarding AI that are certainly applicable to cytology include the need for model validation and continued quality assurance, ethical issues such as the use of patient data in developing algorithms, the need to develop regulatory frameworks regarding what type of data can be utilized and ensuring cybersecurity during data collection and storage, and algorithm development. ***Key Messages:*** While AI will likely play a role in cytology practice in the future, applying this technology to cytology poses a unique set of challenges. A broad understanding of digital pathology and algorithm development is desirable to guide the development of algorithms, as well as the need to be cognizant of potential pitfalls to avoid when incorporating the technology in practice.

Introduction

The incorporation of emerging technologies into pathology is an integral part of contemporary pathology practice. Immunocytochemistry and molecular techniques are examples of such technologies that cytologists have come to embrace as a routine aspect of up-to-date medical care [1]. While these emerging technologies aim to improve patient care and advance the understanding of disease processes, adapting these technologies to a cytopathology-specific context and integrating them into routine practice pose a unique set of challenges that are best resolved using a multidisciplinary approach. Applying artificial intelligence (AI) and machine learning technologies to pathology, and cytopathology in particular, is

karger@karger.com
www.karger.com/acy

Karger

Ewen David McAlpine
Division of Anatomical Pathology
University of the Witwatersrand and National Health Laboratory Service
7 York Road, Parktown 2193 (South Africa)
ewen.mcalpine@wits.ac.za

no different. This review aims to discuss the challenges of implementing deep learning in cytopathology practice.

The terms AI, machine learning, and deep learning are often used interchangeably by newcomers to this field of computer science. This, together with a lack of acquaintance with machine learning jargon, can lead to misunderstanding between computer scientists and cytologists. AI is a broad, overarching term used to describe techniques that allow a computer to mimic human behavior by following a set of rules. The term AI incorporates machine learning and deep learning. Machine learning techniques allow a computer to "learn" from data without being explicitly programmed. Deep learning extrapolates the idea of machine learning by allowing algorithms to train themselves by exposing neural networks to large quantities of data [2]. Furthermore, machine learning methods can be divided into supervised learning, unsupervised learning, and reinforcement learning. Supervised learning requires algorithms to be supplied with data and an expected output (called a *label*) that the algorithm is trained to predict. The process of annotating/labeling data can be an extremely time-consuming and laborious task for cytologists [3]. Unsupervised learning explores data without the need for labels by looking for patterns in the data. Reinforcement learning is a branch of machine learning that allows algorithms to explore ways to solve problems using a reward-based system, where the algorithm attempts to maximize its reward [2]. The most common algorithms cytology personnel will encounter in a diagnostic setting are likely to be supervised learning techniques. Supervised learning algorithms include (i) classification algorithms, where the computer is trained to predict a label (e.g., the presence or absence of malignant cells in an image), and (ii) regression algorithms, where a model predicts a numerical value (e.g., expected patient survival time, given a set of input features) [4].

Digital Cytology

Utilizing a digital workflow in pathology practice has become possible in recent years due to advances in whole slide scanning technology with the development of high-capacity, high-speed slide scanners, although digital workflows are not yet universal in cytology practice [5]. Implementing whole slide imaging in cytology does, however, result in a new set of challenges for this technology. Briefly, these cytology-specific challenges include (i) the 3-dimensional distribution of cytology material on a glass slide (e.g., cell clusters), resulting in the need for capturing images on different focal planes (*z*-stacking), which leads to increased image acquisition time and larger file sizes; (ii) the large amounts of color information (i.e., multiple staining techniques, e.g., Papanicolaou and Romanowsky stains); and (iii) lack of anatomical orientation and information at multiple image scales (different magnifications) [5–7].

Cytology imaging systems have been in existence for 25 years and are primarily for screening of cervical smears. The ThinPrep Imaging System and FocalPoint GS Imaging System both have FDA approval. These systems both use algorithms applied to glass slides that are scanned in using these imaging systems. These are not fully automated but rather detect areas of the smear that are most likely to be abnormal and present these to the cytologist who must then decide if they are truly abnormal or not. The FocalPoint does have a feature whereby the 20% of glass slides that are least likely to contain an abnormality can be archived without further review [8]. Several studies have shown these imaging systems to be as sensitive as manual screening in detecting cervical lesions, as well as allowing smears to be screened faster, improving productivity as more smears can be screened daily [9]. However, a large trial in England that looked at both systems concluded that they were not as sensitive as manual screening although productivity was enhanced [10]. Despite the increased productivity of cytologists, it has been shown that a cytologist utilizing one of these imagers will start performing suboptimally if screening >100 slides per day [11]. Thrall [9], in a review of automation of Pap smear screening published in 2019 concluded that "research into automated screening continues but so far technology has failed to revolutionize screening in the way that has long been predicted."

The implementation of AI algorithms in cytology is greatly enabled by a digital workflow and instituting a digital workflow may be the first hurdle that needs to be overcome when implementing deep learning in cytology. There are several aspects related to the image acquisition of cytology material (e.g., overlapping cells, cellular degeneration, poor focus, and artifacts) that may impair digital datasets, thereby making it challenging to train algorithms (Fig. 1). In addition, WSI and software packages need to be calibrated and maintained in line with all laboratory equipment [12].

In addition to WSI, laboratories will need to ensure that computer monitors employed to view scanned slides are of sufficient quality in terms of color, image resolution, and size. Laboratories will also need to be able to

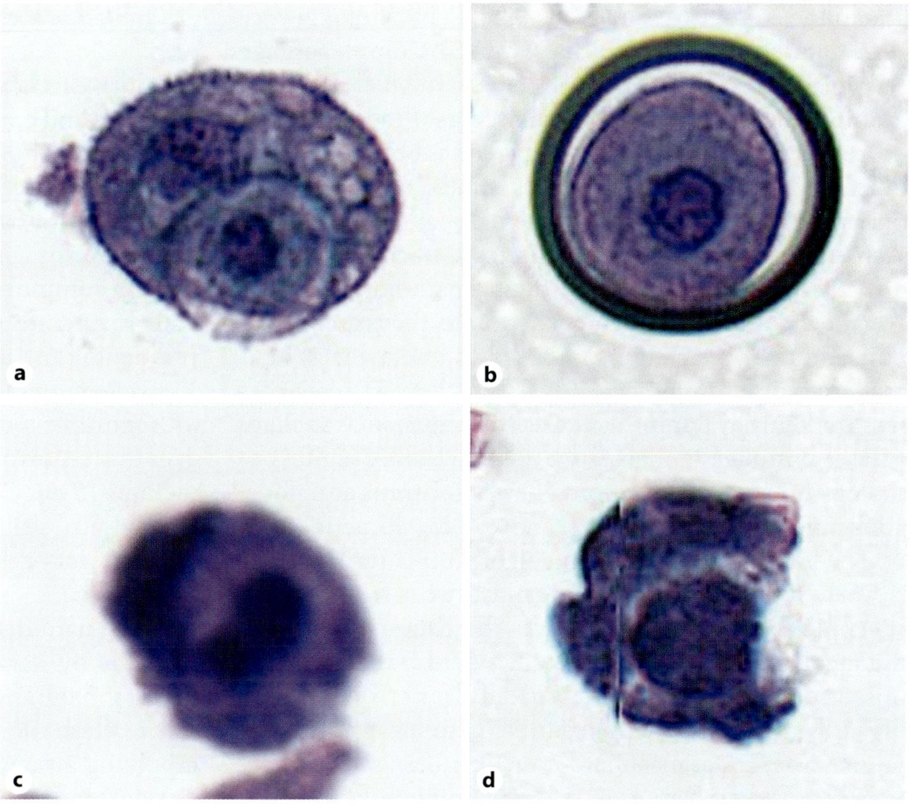

Fig. 1. Different cytologic features that make training deep learning algorithms challenging. **a** Overlapping cells make it difficult for cell classifiers to segment individual cells. **b** Air bubble artifact that may hamper cell detection. **c** Degenerated cell that was scanned in one *z*-plane out of focus lacks sufficient features to be reliably analyzed. **d** Image stitching artifact is shown, which may unnecessarily contribute to increased cell/nuclear irregularity measurements (ThinPrep, Pap stain).

store images with laboratory information systems available for easy and quick transfer of images from storage to individual monitors [12]. This may require substantial investment in laboratory IT infrastructure.

Added Responsibility for Cytologists

Ensuring that cytologists do not impede the implementation of deep learning in cytology is of paramount importance and implementing AI in cytology will place added responsibility on cytologists [13]. Cytologists need to place themselves at the center of the development and validation of these technologies in cytology [1]. Moreover, they need to have a basic understanding of AI technologies, how these techniques are implemented in cytology practice, and how these methods are evaluated, validated, and regulated [14, 15]. As already alluded to above, a major hurdle to overcome in this process is to narrow the knowledge gap between cytologists and machine learning experts [16]. This knowledge gap is not only because of the cytologist, as machine learning experts are unlikely to understand some of the nuances of cytology and will accordingly need to rely on cytologists as *domain experts*[17]. According to Aeffner et al. [12], pathologists (and by extension cytologists) will need to ensure that the algorithm is detecting what is meant to be detected, recognizing the relevant cells and ensuring that the data generated are relevant and significant.

AI technologies have enormous potential benefits for cytology and knowledge of this potential may motivate cytologists to embrace this emerging technology. Automation of mundane, often time-consuming tasks (e.g., screening Ziehl-Neelsen stains for acid-fast bacilli), virtual peer review, and more abstract uses such as identifying previously unknown visual features are some of the potential applications of AI technology [18].

Availability of Datasets

A challenge common to all machine learning tasks, but also specifically an issue for cytopathology, is the lack of large, high-quality digital datasets on which to train algorithms [4, 18]. Deep learning algorithms traditionally require large amounts of high-quality annotated data, and due to the complexity of the visual data in cytology, very large datasets may be required [3, 4, 18]. Complex image classification tasks may require datasets of several million examples for training to achieve acceptable accuracy [4]. Moreover, annotation of cytology data is best performed by expert cytologists [18], which is a time-consuming task that places an additional burden on an already constrained profession. A few pathology teaching sets are now online. However, many digital pathology datasets are not widely available, and, if available, they can only be utilized under restrictions imposed by the owners, be it academic or commercial [19]. Given the vast resources required for developing a dataset, the reluctance to share datasets is understandable, but this will hinder digital pathology in terms of developing new algorithms and novel application of this technology in pathology practice.

The goal of a deep learning algorithm is for the algorithm to perform well on real-world, unseen data (termed *generalization*), and this requires the data used to train the algorithm to be as representative as possible of the unseen data. Good quality data ideally lack errors in labeling and are unbiased with regard to extreme examples or outliers [4]. Datasets should contain sufficient diversity to account for variation in color, staining, artifacts, and cytologic features and should contain examples captured using multiple different devices and on samples derived from multiple laboratories on different days of the week and prepared by different technologists [3, 20].

The term *overfitting* refers to an algorithm that performs well on training data but does not generalize to unseen, real-world data. This can be caused by a model that is too complex for the task, which allows the model to learn irrelevant features, a dataset that is of insufficient quantity or a dataset that is not representative of real-world data [2, 4]. Similarly, a model that is too simple for the task will be unable to learn from the data and will *underfit* in a real-world setting [4].

A commonly used technique to test the ability of an algorithm to generalize is to set aside a portion of the dataset specifically for algorithm evaluation. Ideally, a dataset is split into 3 parts: a training set, a validation set, and a test set [2]. The algorithm is trained on the training set, evaluated on the validation set during tuning of the algorithm, and then finally tested on the unseen test set when the algorithm is ready for deployment [2].

Furthermore, when one employs a cytologist's annotation as the gold standard for algorithm training, this may result in the so-called "gold-standard paradox", where the algorithm's output may, in fact, be more accurate and reproducible than the cytologists labeling the data [3].

Challenges with Algorithm Training

Enormous computer resources, both in terms of storage space and computing power, are required for deploying digital pathology coupled with AI in clinical practice. This includes both the storage space and computing power required for deep learning algorithm development and training. This, in turn, means that a significant investment in computer infrastructure and individuals with the skills to operate and maintain this are needed to develop and deploy these algorithms [3]. As already mentioned, digitization of cytology slides at high magnification and with multiple focal planes (z-stacking) results in large file sizes that require safe, secure storage ideally with multiple backups [5, 6]. Compression of digitized whole slide images may be utilized in an attempt to reduce size of the scanned image. However, this may lead to loss of information [12].

Training a deep learning model with millions of parameters by iterating over a training dataset is called a *training loop* and is currently the fundamental way in which these models are developed [2]. This process of supplying a network with data, allowing it to make predictions on the data, calculating the error between these predictions and the truth and updating the model's parameters (*weights*) accordingly (in a process called *backpropagation*) requires a large amount of computing power [2]. More specifically, multiple graphics processing units (GPUs) are required, and these can be expensive [2–4]. GPUs do, however, greatly improve training times; AI-based models that will take days or weeks to train on a traditional computer's central processing unit can take just a few hours on a dedicated GPU [4]. While cloud-based GPU-equipped virtual machines are available for hire (e.g., Amazon Web Services, Google Cloud, and Microsoft Azure), these also come at a cost and may not be ideal for a medical setting as medical data need to be properly curated and secured at all times [4][4]. Moreover, processing visual cytopathology data (e.g., whole slide images) may be more computationally intensive than other computer vision tasks due to the very large size, proprietary file formats and complexity of the visual data involved [18]. Network speeds also require consideration when implementing AI technologies in cytopathology. Depending on specific workflow configurations, large whole slide images will initially need to be transferred from the whole slide scanner to a storage location, and these may again need to be transferred to a different image processing environment [3].

Cytologists will also need to play a critical role in determining what kinds of algorithms are developed for cytopathology practice. One of the potentials of deep learning is that it is able to learn associations from data without being explicitly trained how to do this by a human observer. This means that deep learning algorithms may be able to make use of morphological characteristics previously unknown to cytologists; however, a lack of interpretability by cytologists is likely to elicit distrust by the professional community. To mitigate against this, algorithms could be trained to reproduce currently accepted cytopathology classification schemes (e.g., The Paris System for Urine Cytology) [21]. As an example of this, replication of an existing classification scheme has been proposed for urine cytology [22]. This approach further illustrates the fact that more than 1 deep learning algorithm may be required to fulfill this approach; this use of multiple, sequential algorithms is termed a *pipeline*. Another challenge when building an algorithm for cytopathology is to determine what cytology material to use. Designing an AI-based algorithm to screen a slide with a liquid-based preparation and a Papanicolaou stain will be very different from a tool that analyzes direct smears with a Diff-Quik stain.

Understanding how an algorithm's performance is evaluated is also of paramount importance [13]. Commonly used metrics to assess algorithm performance include *accuracy*, *precision*, and *recall*, and the specific setting in which an algorithm will be employed is critical to understanding which of these metrics one should attempt to maximize when training an algorithm. These metrics are calculated from the well-known *confusion matrix* that have been elucidated previously [13].

AI-based algorithms also use the *receiver operating characteristic* (ROC) curve to measure their performance. This is a popular metric of evaluation because it quickly provides a visual illustration of algorithm performance. An example of an ROC curve is provided in Figure 2 [22]. The ROC curve plots recall (i.e., sensitivity or true-positive rate) against 1 – specificity (i.e., the false-positive rate) [4]. The dashed line in Figure 2 represents a purely random classifier and a good classifier attempts to stay as close to the top left-hand corner of the graph as possible [4]. One can also measure the area under the curve of the ROC curve. The higher the area under the curve of ROC, the better the model is at accurately predicting or distinguishing between cases with/without a specific pathology diagnosis.

When selecting the evaluation metrics to be used, one must consider the effect of false positives and negatives

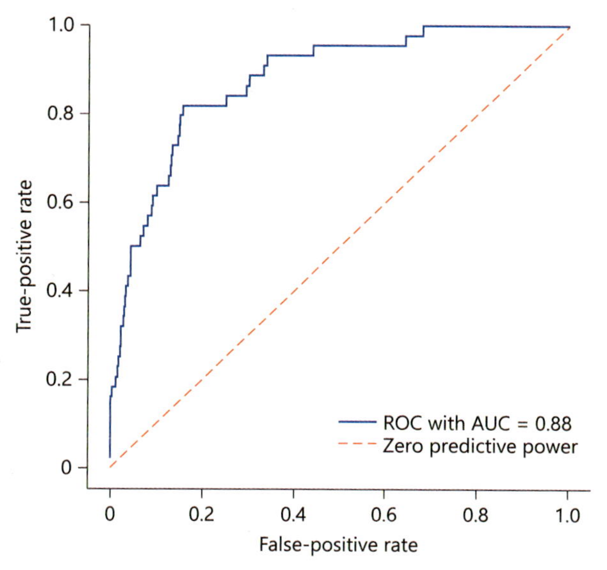

Fig. 2. An example of a receiver operating characteristic (ROC) curve – used with permission [22].

produced by the algorithm and the consequences of these errors in a diagnostic setting [23]. This decision is also likely to be guided by the intended use of the algorithm: for algorithms designed to screen for the presence of an abnormality (e.g., cervical screening), a high recall (sensitivity) and lower specificity are most appropriate, while the opposite is true for algorithms designed to screen out normal specimens (e.g., urine cytology in symptomatic patients) [14]. Accuracy is not an ideal measure for use in a cytopathology setting, as it does not distinguish between the type of errors (false positives or false negatives) made by the algorithm [24].

Challenges Using Algorithms in Routine Practice

As with any new technology, end users (i.e., cytologists), clinicians, and patients may not trust these algorithms initially. In AI, this issue is further aggravated by the fact that many deep learning algorithms are opaque to human understanding [3]. This is termed the "black box problem" by most authors and relates to the "lack of transparency, explainability, and provability" [3] of an algorithm's output to human observers [18]. Efforts to improve the interpretability of these algorithms to a human observer can result in diminished algorithm performance

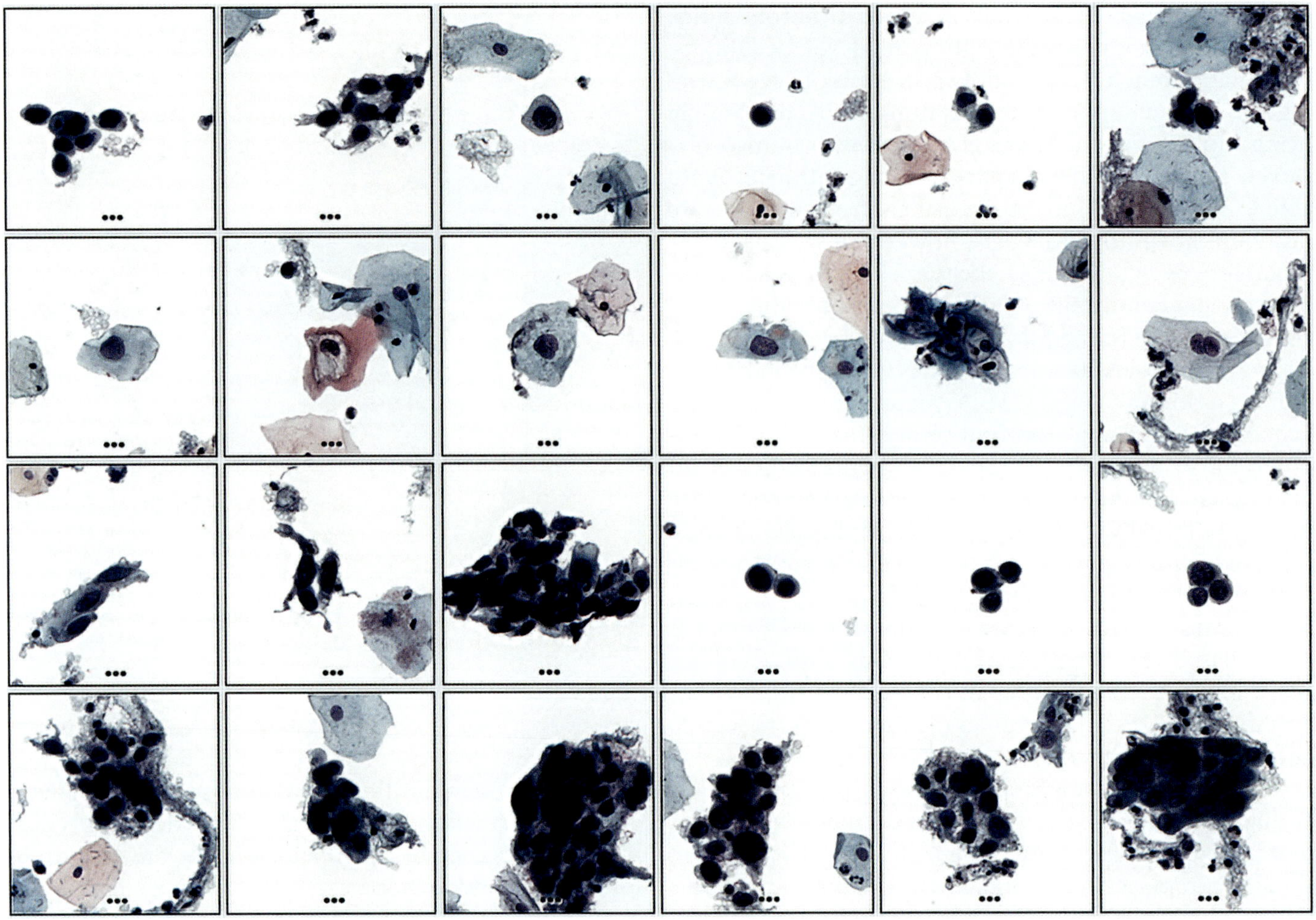

Fig. 3. Image gallery display from Hologic's digital cytology system in development for computer-assisted screening of Pap tests showing multiple image patches of squamous cells from a ThinPrep Pap test with mostly features of high-grade squamous intraepithelial lesion – used with permission.

[6]. Examples of converting the AI output into explainable formats for human digestion are overlaying heatmaps on pathology images (often color coordinated to match probability), or displaying high-ranking image patches on a computer monitor in the form of an image gallery (Fig. 3).

Ideally, any algorithm incorporated into a new workflow should have minimal or no detrimental impact on current workflows and efficiencies, and be simple to use for cytologists [25, 26]. This may require that the algorithm accommodate cases being first screened by cytotechnologists and then subsequently reviewed by pathologists. In addition, incorporating AI technology in a cytopathology workflow would have to translate to non-inferior patient outcome or perhaps even an improved patient outcome and even a return on investment made by laboratories such as improved turnaround time and cost savings [18]. Griffin and Treanor [27] undertook a small study contrasting viewing glass slides with a microscope and viewing digital slides and found that digital slides were 67% less efficient. Reasons for this included that the digital viewer afforded a smaller field of view, there were problems with the software designs utilized for viewing the slides, and participants lacked training and experience [27]. Other studies have confirmed limitations of equipment and suboptimal image resolution as downsides in digital pathology [28].

Current AI technologies, such as neural networks, are mostly considered "weak AI" in that they perform well on a specific task (otherwise known as *uni-task orientation*) but are unable to compare to a human's ability to multitask or think laterally (i.e., "strong AI") [18]. Additionally, classification algorithms typically output Boolean values (e.g., true/false, presence/absence), which is an oversimplification of the nuances of a cytology diagnosis, which makes use of human cognition, understanding of clinical context, and practitioner experience to render a diagnosis [18].

Challenges around Model Validation and Continuing Quality Assurance

Any software deployed in a diagnostic setting is considered an instance of *software as a medical device* (SaMD) and, as such, AI algorithms deployed in a cytopathology setting will need to undergo analytical and clinical validation, as well as receive possible regulatory approval [15]. The process by which this validation occurs is stipulated by the International Medical Device Regulators Forum [29]. In addition, countries and different institutions will have their own regulatory frameworks and requirements to achieve before permitting an algorithm to be implemented in routine diagnostics.

Developers of AI algorithms intended for deployment in cytopathology will need to collect data on the algorithm's performance metrics (e.g., accuracy, specificity, and sensitivity), as well as the algorithm's limitations prior to deployment [29]. Following deployment, manufacturers will need to monitor the algorithm's performance in a real-world setting – including performance metrics and safety data [29].

Kim et al. [30] demonstrated that most published literature reporting the performance of AI in medical image analysis were "proof-of-concept" studies that did not employ methodology recommended to validate real-world performance of these algorithms. Recommendations for studies designed to evaluate the clinical performance of AI technology for medical image analysis include prospective, multi-institutional study design that enrolls patients/samples that meet specified inclusion criteria adequately describing the target population in a consecutive manner [31]. Prospective study design should reduce the risk of dataset bias [31]. In contrast to algorithm training, where large quantities of data are needed for training, clinical validation will require less, but sufficiently representative, data, although further research into the exact number of cases required for clinical validation is required [31].

Following model deployment in a clinical setting, cytologists will need to ensure appropriate and ongoing quality assurance of these algorithms; however, there is currently no agreement of how this is best achieved. It may be advisable that all glass slides in these types of trials undergo review by a third party, in addition to comparing the diagnosis of the glass and digital slide, to adjust for interobserver variability [27]. Williams et al. [32] suggest that a small set of appropriate glass slides be collected for both the algorithm and cytologists to view daily for several weeks to document the algorithm's reproducibility to ensure that the algorithm's outputs are reliable for clinical practice. Guidelines for validation and ongoing quality control are required to promote widespread and safe adoption for clinical use.

Concerns around Ethics, Privacy, and Cybersecurity

Global ethical principles, as well as national and/or local regulations, need to be developed regarding the appropriate use of patient data in developing AI algorithms. This involves matters such as patient consent, data ownership, and storage and possible transfer of data to third parties such as commercial companies in order to develop algorithms. A balance needs to be found between financial viability of entities developing algorithms and the need to ensure that the benefits of AI can be experienced by society as a whole and not confined to just those communities served by institutions that can afford to purchase expensive digital pathology platforms [3]. According to Mazer et al. [19], the glass slide can be viewed by many people using a variety of existing microscopes. This is in contrast to WSI whereby these imagers are manufactured by a few companies and may not be within financial reach of many laboratories especially in low middle income countries [19].

Mazer et al. [19] propose the formation of a "digital commons" whereby WSI are housed in a non-proprietary format with pathologists and institutions able to access these datasets under realistic conditions. Furthermore, new ideas and hypotheses resulting from these datasets should be made accessible to others working in the field. However, these authors do acknowledge that absence of a profit incentive may thwart innovation. This dilemma is not only confined to pathology. Davies et al. [33] state that authors involved in 3D digital datasets of biological and paleontological specimens do not regularly publish their supporting information. This means that outcomes cannot readily be verified nor further studies by other researchers undertaken [33]. They recommend that agreement among authors, repositories, journal editors, peer reviewers, and funding agencies be reached in order to fully utilize the potential of digital datasets.

To keep up to date with new theories and practices in medicine, algorithms will require regular updates. It needs to be determined if users will be compelled to pay for these updates. If a laboratory is unable to pay for or install new updates, this could lead to a situation whereby patients are diagnosed using outdated algorithms [34].

It is necessary to develop regulatory frameworks to determine when data can be used without explicit patient consent (even if patient data are anonymized), and what type of data can be shared and utilized to develop algorithms [35]. Legal institutions, bioethicists, and other relevant groups will need to be consulted in this regard. An advantage of using cytology images in digital pathology is that no patient identifiers are present, unlike histopathology in which identifiers such as tattoos may be seen. Nonetheless, before cytology images can be utilized, permission (patient or institutional) has to be sought. In addition, cybersecurity must be ensured during data collection and storage and transfer of patient data from a health institution to a third party who will develop the algorithm [36]. These issues become more complicated when dealing with adaptive commercial algorithms, which continually change and improve over time by consuming and learning from growing datasets. The use of adaptive algorithms necessitates evaluation of the need for applications to necessary regulatory bodies and repeat validation in a clinical setting [15].

It is vital that users of AI understand its limitations including false negatives and false positives. False negatives would be the failure of the AI system to detect what it should be identifying, while false-positive results may bring about unnecessary procedures that are costly to both the patient and health care system [36]. An AI system that surpasses human cytologists may not, on further interrogation, be beneficial. This is due to the potential detection of inconsequential lesions [37]. When Scotland introduced screening for prostatic carcinoma, for example, there was an increased detection of malignancy without a commensurate reduction in mortality. This may have been due, in part, to uncovering latent malignancies that might never have become symptomatic [38]. One must be aware that this could be the case with AI-based tools that are too sensitive.

Conclusion

As the utilization of AI becomes more widespread, cytologists need to be at the forefront of algorithm development to ensure that the algorithms created meet the needs of the cytology discipline. While there certainly are advantages to the introduction of AI, cytologists have to be cognizant of the challenges when developing, implementing, interacting with, and overseeing deep learning algorithms. A broad understanding of digital pathology and AI is desirable in order to guide those developing algorithms as to what is required as well as alerting them as to what pitfalls to avoid. Perception of algorithm limitations will help ensure their optimal performance when these AI tools are employed by a laboratory.

Conflict of Interest Statement

E.D.M. and P.M.M. have no conflicts of interest to declare. L.P. is on the Medical Advisory Board for Ibex and a consultant for Hamamatsu.

Funding Sources

The authors did not receive any funding.

Author Contributions

E.D.M., P.M.M., and L.P. all contributed to the writing and editing of the manuscript.

References

1 Salto-Tellez M, Maxwell P, Hamilton P. Artificial intelligence: the third revolution in pathology. Histopathology. 2019 Feb [cited 2019 Mar 24];74(3):372–6.
2 Chollet F. Deep learning with python. 1st ed. Greenwich, CT: Manning Publications Co.; 2017.
3 Abels E, Pantanowitz L, Aeffner F, Zarella MD, vd Laak J, Bui MM, et al. Computational pathology definitions, best practices, and recommendations for regulatory guidance: a white paper from the Digital Pathology Association. J Pathol. 2019;249(3):286–94.
4 Géron A. Hands-on machine learning with scikit-learn, keras & tensorFlow. 2nd ed. O'Reilly Media Inc.; 2019. p. 23–32.
5 Capitanio A, Dina RE, Treanor D. Digital cytology: a short review of technical and methodological approaches and applications. Cytopathology. 2018;29(4):317–25.

6 Niazi MKK, Parwani AV, Gurcan MN. Digital pathology and artificial intelligence. Lancet Oncol. 2019;20(5):e253–61.
7 Gill G. Cytopreparation: principles & practice. New York: Springer; 2013. Vols. 143–188; p. 217–43.
8 Levi AW, Chhieng DC, Schofield K, Kowalski D, Harigopal M. Implementation of FocalPoint GS location-guided imaging system: experience in a clinical setting. Cancer Cytopathol. 2012 Apr;120(2):126–33.
9 Thrall MJ. Automated screening of Papanicolaou tests: a review of the literature. Diagn Cytopathol. 2019 Jan;47(1):20–7.
10 Kitchener HC, Blanks R, Dunn G, Gunn L, Desai M, Albrow R, et al. Automation-assisted versus manual reading of cervical cytology (MAVARIC): a randomised controlled trial. Lancet Oncol. 2011 Jan;12(1):56–64.
11 Levi AW, Galullo P, Gordy K, Mikolaiski N, Schofield K, Elsheikh TM, et al. Increasing cytotechnologist workload above 100 slides per day using the BD focalpoint GS imaging system negatively affects screening performance. Am J Clin Pathol. 2012 Dec;138(6):811–5.
12 Aeffner F, Adissu HA, Boyle MC, Cardiff RD, Hagendorn E, Hoenerhoff MJ, et al. Digital microscopy, image analysis, and virtual slide repository. ILAR J. 2018;59(1):66.
13 McAlpine ED, Michelow P. The cytopathologist's role in developing and evaluating artificial intelligence in cytopathology practice. Cytopathology. Blackwell Publishing Ltd; 2020.
14 Rubin DL. Artificial intelligence in imaging: the radiologist's role. J Am Coll Radiol. 2019; 16(9 Pt B):1309–17.
15 FDA. Proposed Regulatory Framework for Modifications to Artificial Intelligence/Machine Learning (AI/ML)-Based Software as a Medical Device (SaMD). 2019;1–20. Available from: https://www.fda.gov/downloads/MedicalDevices/DigitalHealth/SoftwareasaMedicalDevice/UCM635052.pdf.
16 Panesar A. Machine learning and AI for healthcare: big data for improved health outcomes. Berkeley, CA: Apress; 2019.
17 Casey K. 2019: https://enterprisersproject.com/article/2019/6/how-staff-ai-team-11-key-roles.
18 Tizhoosh HR, Pantanowitz L. Artificial intelligence and digital pathology: challenges and opportunities. J Pathol Inform. 2018;9(1):38. http://www.jpathinformatics.org/text.asp?2018/9/1/38/245402.http://dx.doi.org/10.4103/jpi.jpi_53_18.
19 Mazer BL, Paulson N, Sinard JH. Protecting the pathology commons in the digital era. Arch Pathol Lab Med. 2020 Jun;144(9):1037–40.
20 Marée R. The need for careful data collection for pattern recognition in digital pathology. J Pathol Inform. 2017 [cited 2018 Dec 2];8:19. http://www.jpathinformatics.org/text.asp?2017/8/1/19/204200.http://dx.doi.org/10.4103/jpi.jpi_94_16.
21 Barkan GA, Wojcik EM, Nayar R, Savic-Prince S, Quek ML, Kurtycz DF, et al. The Paris System for reporting urinary cytology: the quest to develop a standardized terminology. Acta Cytol. 2016 [cited 2018 Dec 2]; 60(3):185–97.
22 Sanghvi AB, Allen EZ, Callenberg KM, Pantanowitz L. Performance of an artificial intelligence algorithm for reporting urine cytopathology. Cancer Cytopathol. 2019 Oct 1; 127(10):658–66.
23 Panesar A. Machine learning and AI for healthcare: big data for improved health outcomes. Berkeley, CA: Apress; 2019.
24 Japkowicz N. Why Question Machine Learning Evaluation Methods? (An illustrative review of the shortcomings of current methods). In: The AAAI Conference on Artificial Intelligence [Internet]. 2006. p. 6–11. Available from: https://aaai.org/.
25 Landau MS, Pantanowitz L. Artificial intelligence in cytopathology: a review of the literature and overview of commercial landscape. J Am Soc Cytopathol. 2019;8(4):230–41.
26 Ngiam KY, Khor IW. Big data and machine learning algorithms for health-care delivery. Lancet Oncol. 2019;20(5):e262–73.
27 Griffin J, Treanor D. Digital pathology in clinical use: where are we now and what is holding us back? Histopathology. Blackwell Publishing Ltd; 2017. Vol. 70; p. 134–45.
28 Araújo ALD, Arboleda LPA, Palmier NR, Fonsêca JM, de Pauli Paglioni M, Gomes-Silva W, et al. The performance of digital microscopy for primary diagnosis in human pathology: a systematic review. Virchows archiv. Springer Verlag; 2019. Vol. 474; p. 269–87.
29 IMDRF SaMD Working Group. Software as a Medical Device (SaMD): clinical evaluation. Int Med Device Regul Forum. 2017 Sep:4–8.
30 Kim DW, Jang HY, Kim KW, Shin Y, Park SH. Design characteristics of studies reporting the performance of artificial intelligence algorithms for diagnostic analysis of medical images: results from recently published papers. Korean J Radiol. 2019 Mar;20(3):405–10.
31 Park SH, Han K. Methodologic guide for evaluating clinical performance and effect of artificial intelligence technology for medical diagnosis and prediction. Radiology. Radiological Society of North America Inc.; 2018. Vol. 286; p. 800–9.
32 Williams BJ, Knowles C, Treanor D. Maintaining quality diagnosis with digital pathology: a practical guide to ISO 15189 accreditation. J Clin Pathol. 2019 Oct [cited 2019 Oct 22];72(10):663–8. http://jcp.bmj.com/lookup/doi/10.1136/jclinpath-2019-205944. http://dx.doi.org/10.1136/jclinpath-2019-205944.
33 Davies TG, Rahman IA, Lautenschlager S, Cunningham JA, Asher RJ, Barrett PM, et al. Open data and digital morphology. Proc Biol Sci. 2017 Apr;284(1852):20170194.
34 Prabhu SP. Ethical challenges of machine learning and deep learning algorithms. The lancet oncology. Lancet Publishing Group; 2019. Vol. 20; p. 621–2.
35 Turnquist C, Roberts-Gant S, Hemsworth H, White K, Browning L, Rees G, et al. On the edge of a digital pathology transformation: views from a cellular pathology laboratory focus group. J Pathol Inform. 2019 Jan 1;10(1):37.
36 Jaremko JL, Azar M, Bromwich R, Lum A, Alicia Cheong LH, Gibert M, et al. Canadian Association of Radiologists white paper on ethical and legal issues related to artificial intelligence in radiology. Canadian Association of Radiologists Journal. Canadian Medical Association; 2019. Vol. 70; p. 107–18.
37 Huss R, Coupland SE. Software-assisted decision support in digital histopathology. J Pathol. 2020 Feb 25;250(5):685–92.
38 Brewster DH, Fraser LA, Harris V, Black RJ. Rising incidence of prostate cancer in Scotland: increased risk or increased detection? BJU Int. 2000;85(4):463–3.

Review

Acta Cytologica

Acta Cytologica 2021;65:310–323
DOI: 10.1159/000510992

Received: June 9, 2020
Accepted: August 19, 2020
Published online: November 11, 2020

Recent Advances in Medical Image Processing

Zhen Huang Qiang Li Ju Lu Junlin Feng Jiajia Hu Ping Chen

Hangzhou Zhiwei Information and Technology Inc., Hangzhou, China

Keywords
Medical imaging · Convolution neural network · Deep learning · Artificial intelligence

Abstract
Background: Application and development of the artificial intelligence technology have generated a profound impact in the field of medical imaging. It helps medical personnel to make an early and more accurate diagnosis. Recently, the deep convolution neural network is emerging as a principal machine learning method in computer vision and has received significant attention in medical imaging. ***Key Message:*** In this paper, we will review recent advances in artificial intelligence, machine learning, and deep convolution neural network, focusing on their applications in medical image processing. To illustrate with a concrete example, we discuss in detail the architecture of a convolution neural network through visualization to help understand its internal working mechanism. ***Summary:*** This review discusses several open questions, current trends, and critical challenges faced by medical image processing and artificial intelligence technology.

Introduction

The medical imaging technology plays a key role in a wide range of clinical examinations and procedures, and traditionally most of the interpretation of medical images is carried out by physicians and medical experts. Artificial intelligence (AI) and deep learning have made significant progress in computer vision in the last few years and achieved human-level classification performance on various object recognition tasks [1–3]. Naturally, a lot of research work focuses on applying and adapting deep learning methods to clinical workflow including disease diagnostics and recommendations for patient treatment. Specifically, deep learning and AI can assist medical experts to make a more thorough and detailed examination, improve quality and efficiency of diagnostics, and reduce the amount of repetitive work so they can focus on more critical aspects of patient care.

AI as a research field started in the 1950s from the field of computer science, and early work includes McCarthy 1956 with the goal of simulating intelligent behaviors using computers [4]. After moving through several waves of "AI springs" and "AI winters," AI research has recently received significant attention, interest, and investment. Among different research areas in AI, machine learning has made impressive progress in the last decade. Early AI methods were often based on the knowledge of human experts that is expensive to acquire and error prone, or directly models raw image data without any learning of hidden representations.

Modern machine learning techniques, unlike early AI systems, can learn directly from raw data, generate representations needed for tasks at hand, and require little involvement from human experts. Instead, high quality data are essential to machine learning. As the medical in-

karger@karger.com
www.karger.com/acy

Karger

Ping Chen
Department of Engineering, University of Massachusetts
100 William T. Morrissey Blvd.
Boston, MA 02125-3393 (USA)
pineblossom@gmail.com

dustry and hospitals have enormous amounts of data often collected through strict protocols and procedures, machine learning is naturally applied to various medical areas including disease diagnosis, personalized treatment, and drug discovery. Usually data quality and sample size are very important for a machine learning model to acquire sufficient information and make robust predication. For example, the integration of features such as gender, family history, age, weight, and high-risk behaviors plays a critical role in predicting the development of cancer.

With the advances of imaging technology, more detailed low-level information can be obtained. Meanwhile, with more processing power from hardware, the medical imaging technology currently has made significant progress in collecting data for many important clinical domains. Furthermore, image processing methods can play a vital role in numerous medical imaging applications such as image enhancing to augment regions of interest, image segmentation to measure tissue volumes and localize organs, and object recognition to assist diagnosis. Compared to data collected in other domains, a digital medical image is often of high dimension. With engineering and domain expertise, a feature extractor is needed to transform digital image data into feature vectors for the following machine learning model construction as handcrafted features require prohibitive amount of human labor and domain knowledge. As datasets become larger and more complicated (the image dataset ImageNet has >1.2-million images and nearly 1,000 categories [5]), it is not feasible to manually design such feature descriptors that are capable of extracting all the distinguishing features. So, it is logical to let computer self-learn discriminative features without human involvement. Machine learning research communities have developed many useful techniques about this area such as deep belief networks [6, 7], deep neural networks (DNNs) [8], recurrent neural networks [9], and convolution neural networks (CNNs) [1]. These deep learning methods have been applied to many fields including medical imaging analysis [10–12], computer vision [13, 14], and natural language processing [15, 16].

Among these neural network techniques, the most successful model for image analysis is the CNN. The CNN was first introduced by Fukushima [17, 18]. In 1980, LeCun et al. [19] used backpropagation to learn convolution kernel coefficients directly from images of handwritten numbers. The learning process was fully automatic and achieved impressive performance [19, 20]. This approach became the foundation of modern computer vision technology. In the last decade, various CNN architectures have been introduced such as LeNet-5 and shift-invariant neural network. One notable milestone was the contribution of Krizhevsky et al. [1] to ImageNet Challenge in 2012. They proposed a 7-layer CNN (AlexNet) which employed a lot of effective techniques such as ReLU, dropout, and data augmentation. AlexNet achieved significantly better results than the previous state-of-the-art methods. In the following years, more efficient CNN architectures were proposed. Currently, the CNN is used not only in image recognition but also in image detection [21–24], image segmentation [25–27], and image saliency [28].

This overview paper will introduce medical researchers with exciting and important developments in machine learning, deep learning, CNN, and their applications in medical fields. One common critique of machine learning methods is its lack of interpretability and explainability, which is critical in the medical field. We will discuss the interpretation of CNNs in detail. As there exists no theoretical proof on CNNs, we will present some insights from a practical perspective, and medical researchers can adopt machine learning models and results with more confidence and efficacy.

The rest of this paper is organized as follows. In Section 2, we introduce the CNN techniques that have been used for medical image analysis and discuss several methods and open challenges in different application areas. In Section 3, we will discuss CNN architecture in detail. In Section 4, we will explain how to interpret and explain CNN models. We will conclude with a discussion on several critical issues and an outlook for future research trends.

Deep Learning Applications in Medical Image Processing

In this section, we provide an overview of important advances and development of deep learning methods in various medical imaging fields.

Analysis of Digital Pathology Images

Pathology is the study of the causes and effects of diseases, usually through analysis of cell, tissue, and body fluid samples. DNNs have been used in nearly every division of pathology and achieved significant improvement comparing to other analysis methods.

Cytology diagnoses diseases on the cellular level. The CNN has been widely used in the detection and classification of nucleated cells. Combined with Hough transform, the CNN has been applied to localize nucleus centroids [29]. A five-layer CNN was proposed to identify papillary carcinoma on thyroid fine-needle aspiration cytology smears [30]. Unlike the general CNN classification pipeline, where only 1 CNN is developed to recognize nucleated cells, Sanghvi et al. [31] used multiple tiers of CNN models for image classification of urine cytology slides. Six CNNs were trained to detect cell-level features (N/C ratio, hyperchromasia, chromatin coarseness, and nuclear membrane irregularity), and a CNN to identify true cell clusters. All these features were aggregated, and then gradient boosting classifiers were used to make a prediction. The CNN has been used for fluorescently labeled cell segmentation and achieved similar performance with manual annotations [32]. A 16-layer CNN was proposed to analyze parasite-infected red blood cells in blood smears for malaria diagnosis [33]. The CNN was also employed to identify blood cells in medical hyperspectral images [34].

Unlike cytology that mainly focuses on cells, whole slide imaging (WSI) provides quantitative analysis, including measuring size, length, and density of objects and regions. Whole slide tissue images usually have gigapixel-level resolution, and it is computationally expensive to train a CNN on such huge images. Most WSI classification methods extract features on small patches [35–37]. A patch-based CNN model was proposed in [10], and the labels of patches can provide information for cancer subtyping. Then, a new model is trained on histograms of patch-level predictions. The classification results of this method are similar to the interobserver agreement between pathologists. Alternatively, a neural conditional random field (NCRF) was proposed in [38]. The NCRF utilizes spatial correlations between neighboring patches through a fully connected CRF which is directly incorporated on top of a patch-based CNN extractor.

Ophthalmology

One of the early usages of CNN in medical imaging is ophthalmology. Diabetic retinopathy is an eye disorder due to diabetes and may lead to permanent blindness in severe diabetic stages. Diabetic retinopathy can be controlled and treated to delay or reduce vision loss if it is diagnosed at an early stage by the retinal screening test. A CNN model called Inceptionv3 [39] was applied on 2 datasets for the classification between moderate and worst referable diabetic retinopathy [12]. The 2 datasets are Eye Picture Archive Communication System (EyePACS-1) dataset that contains 9,963 images from 4,997 patients and the Messidor-2 dataset that contains 1,748 images from 874 patients. This algorithm achieves high sensitivity and accuracy for detecting referable diabetic retinopathy. Zeng et al. [40] introduced a Siamese-like CNN. It takes binocular fundus images as inputs and learns their correlation to make a prediction.

Radiology

A variety of radiology techniques such as X-rays, computed tomography, magnetic resonance imaging, nuclear medicine, positron emission tomography, and ultrasound are used to diagnose or treat diseases. These techniques usually involve enormous amounts of data. The CNN is a data-driven method. Hence, CNN methods are prevalent in radiology imaging and analysis.

Chest X-rays play a crucial role in the diagnosis of pneumonia. It can show the area of lung inflammation. The CNN is used to detect these areas. A 121-layer CNN model was created that can automatically detect 14 diseases from chest X-rays [11]. They trained the model on ChestX-ray14 dataset released by Wang et al. [41] that contains 112,120 frontal-view X-ray images of 30,805 unique patients. Also, to interpret predictions output by the CNN model, class activation mapping [42] was used to produce heat maps that indicate a certain disease. This model exceeds average radiologist performance on the F1 metric. During COVID-19 pandemic, to quickly detect pneumonia, many radiologists and physicians are actively adopting deep learning methods to augment lung imaging analysis [43–45].

The desired output of many biomedical image applications is the location of cells and/or measurement of object shapes. Those biomedical images include breast ultrasound images, liver tomography images, and brain images. Image segmentation locates and provides pixel-level tagging on objects of interest in biomedical images. Ciresan et al. [46] trained a CNN in a sliding window setup to predict the category label of each pixel by using a local region around the pixel as the input of the CNN. It is time-consuming and has limitations on the region of an object. Ronneberger et al. [47] proposed a CNN called U-Net. U-Net can be treated as an encoder-decoder network, which allows the network to propagate context information to higher resolution layers. Inspired by U-Net, Milletari et al. [48] proposed a CNN architecture called V-net, which learns residuals and improves both accuracy and convergence rate. There are a lot of 3D medical scan image datasets. 3D images display objects at varying depths comparing to a single image in 2D. Images of different depths are correlative to each other. A dual-

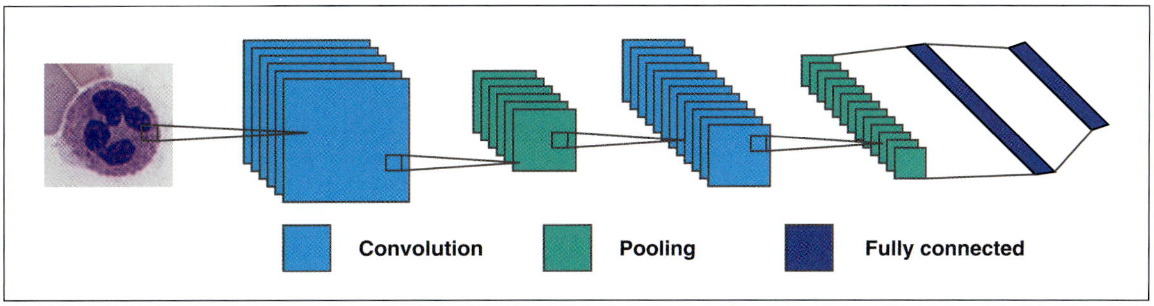

Fig. 1. A convolution neural network, simplified.

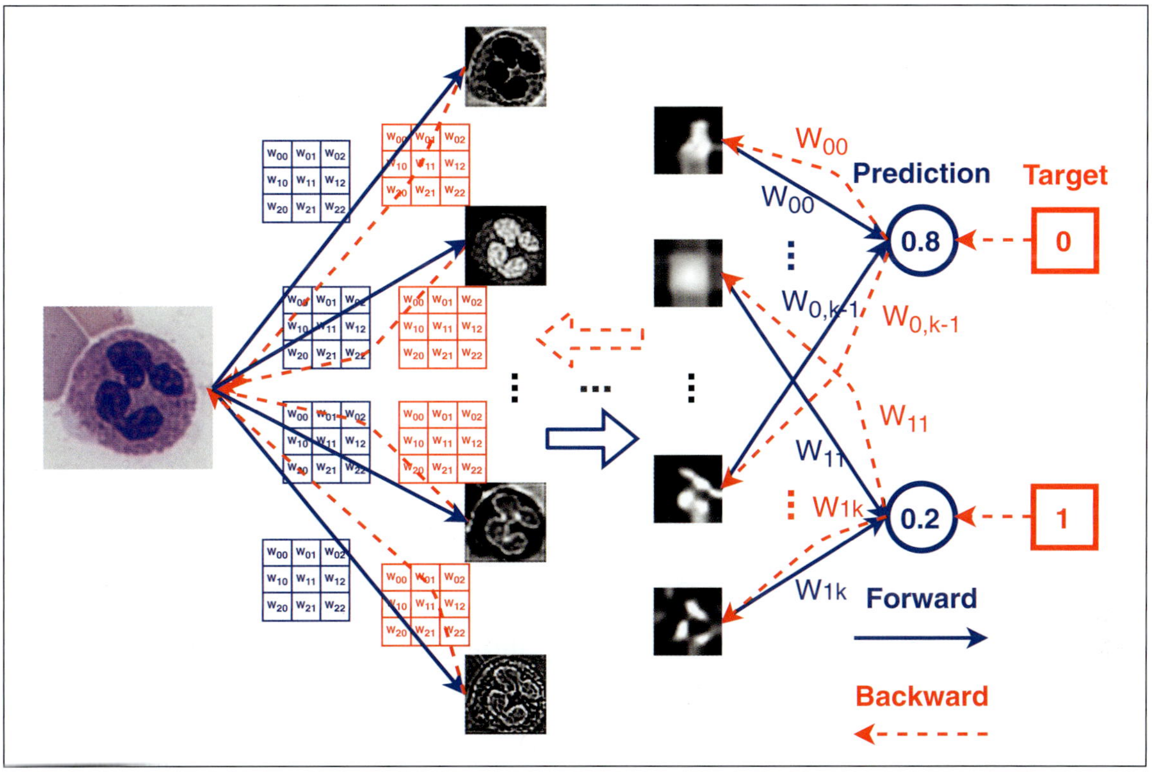

Fig. 2. Illustration of the backpropagation process. The blue arrow denotes the direction of information flow during forward propagation, and red arrow indicates backward propagation of error/loss information. The fully connected nodes link to all elements of feature maps, and weights of fully connected layers (W_{ij}) are a vector.

pathway 3D CNN was introduced for the challenging task of brain lesion segmentation [49]. Neural architecture search (NAS) [50] is a technique for automating the design of CNN. It has been successfully used in large-scale image classification. NAS was used in semantic image segmentation [51]. A hierarchical neural architecture was proposed and attained state-of-art performance without any ImageNet pretraining. After discussing these various medical imaging applications employing deep learning methods, it is clear that the CNN is the most popular model, and we will present the CNN architecture in the next section.

Convolution Neural Network

A general CNN architecture contains convolution layers, pooling layers, and fully connected layers, as shown in Figure 1. In this section, we will first discuss a basic

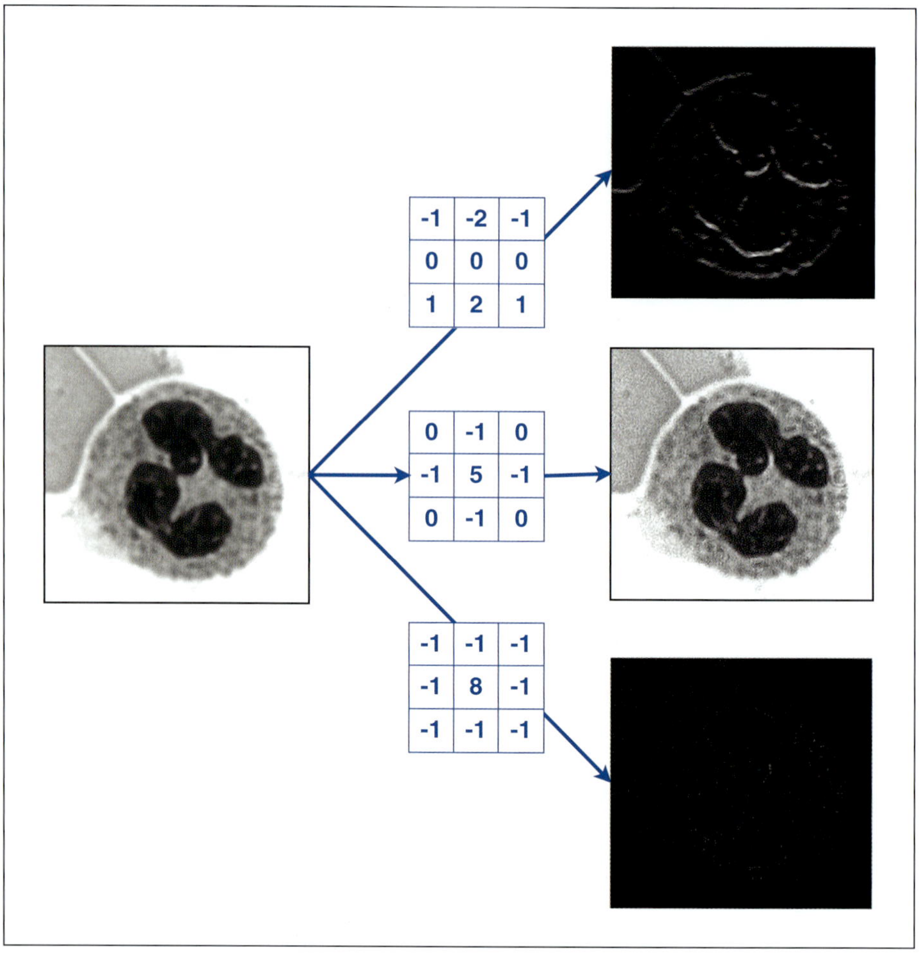

Fig. 3. Examples of effects achievable by different convolution filters including embossing, enhancement, and edge detection.

neural network training method, backpropagation (BP), and then we will present the details of these 3 types of CNN layers.

Backpropagation

The discovery of BP can date back to the 1960s [52]. It became a popular training method for neural networks in 1986 by influential work by Rumelhart et al. [53, 54]. The motivation of BP is to train a multilayered neural network and to learn the mapping of input to output by tuning the parameters of a network. We will use a simple example to illustrate how BP works. A CNN contains 2 convolution layers and 2 fully connected layers. The task is to distinguish neutrophils and lymphocytes. In the beginning, the parameters of a network are randomly assigned. A batch of images of neutrophils and lymphocytes is fed into the network. The last fully connected layer is a vector which has 2 elements. One element represents the probability of being a neutrophil, the other represents the lymphocyte. If the input image is a neutrophil, the expected output of the network should be [0, 1], where 1 is the probability of neutrophils. Otherwise, BP will modify the parameters by calculating the gradient at each parameter based on the chain rule. The output of a network when the input image is a neutrophil will approach to [0, 1] after its parameters have been iterated numerous times. Figure 2 illustrates the whole process. It is worth noting that the target of CNN can also be in other forms. For example, the target can be a matrix when the CNN is used in image segmentation or image saliency (the area of lung inflammation in X-ray images) and can be a coordinate when the CNN is used in object detection (the location information of lesions).

Convolution Layer

One essential part of the CNN is convolution layers that contain multiple convolution filters. A convolution filter is used to modify or enhance an image by emphasiz-

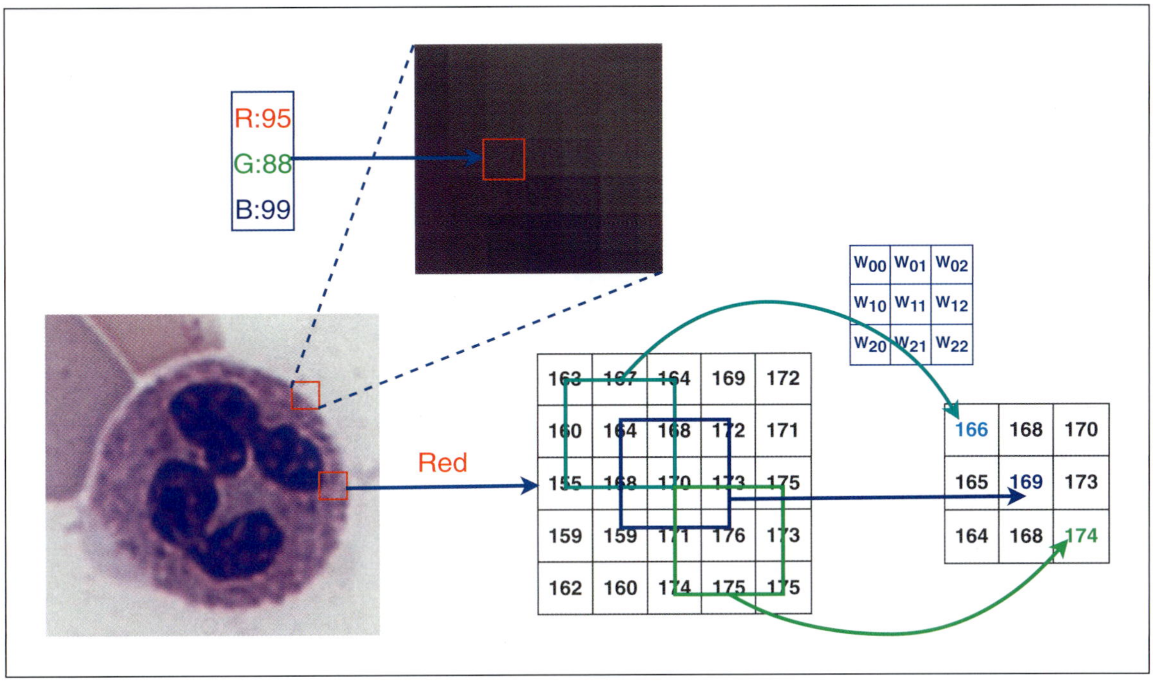

Fig. 4. Illustration of convolution in a 5 × 5 image with a 3 × 3 filter. Since convolution operation in each channel of image is the same, only the red channel is shown.

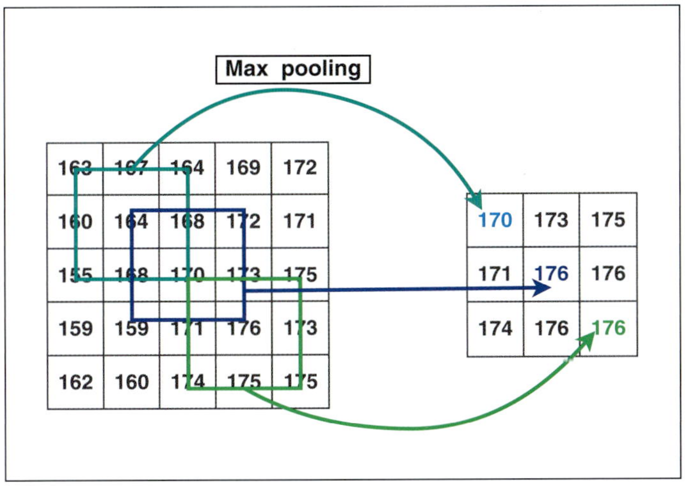

Fig. 5. A pooling example of the pooling layer with max operation.

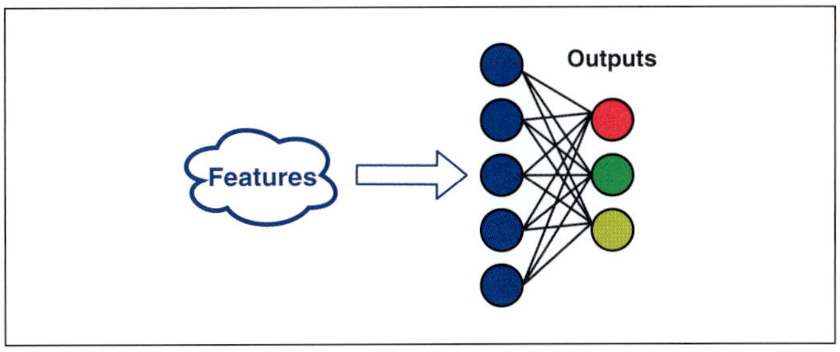

Fig. 6. Illustration of fully connected layers. The features are multiplied by weights and passed through an activation function.

ing or removing certain features in image processing. Those image processing operations include blurring, sharpening, embossing, and edge detection. Depending on the values of the matrix, a filter can cause a wide range of effects, as shown in Figure 3.

An image can be digitized to a matrix. The values of gray scales range from 0 (black) to 255 (white). A color image is just a simple extension of this digitization approach. For example, an RGB image includes red, green, and blue (RGB) channels, so the matrix of an RGB image is 3 dimensional. Image filtering changes the pixel values of an image. As illustrated in Figure 4, the output image is produced by sliding a filter over an input image.

A key property of an image is that neighbor pixels are more strongly correlated than distant pixels. Many image extractors or descriptors [55, 56] extract local features based on small regions of an image. The operation of convolution filters only involves subregions of an image. This mechanism is called local receptive fields [57]. Also, local features that are useful in one region of an image are like-

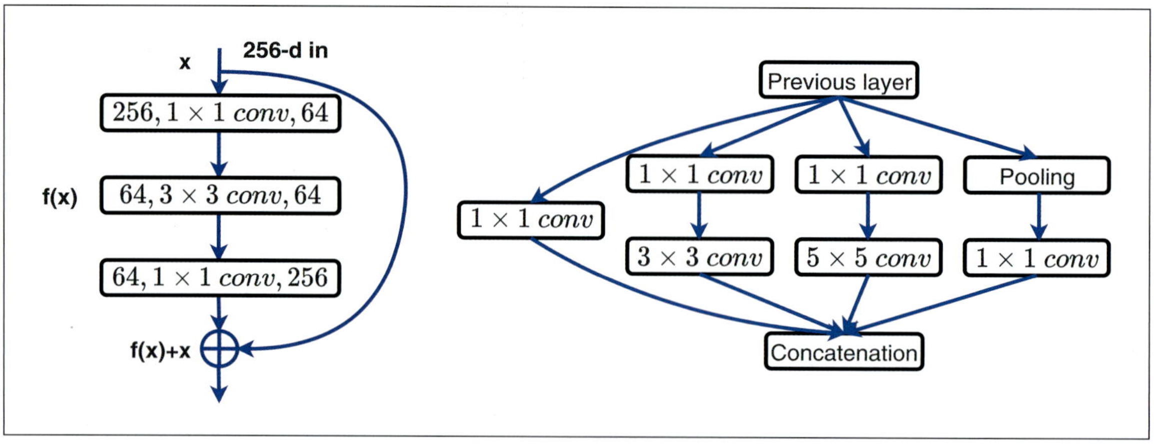

Fig. 7. Left: a block of ResNet with shortcut connections that skips 1 or more layers [3]. Right: an inception module [62]. It becomes not only deeper but also wider.

ly to be useful in other regions of the image, such as granules distributed in white blood cell images. This approach is called weight sharing, which makes CNNs invariant to small shifts and rotations.

Pooling Layer

If an image is resized to half of its size, we can still learn a lot of information from it. As shown in [58, 59], medical images contain significant local and global redundancy, so it is reasonable to compress features of an image in the CNN. One of the image compression methods used in the CNN is pooling layer that is a form of nonlinear downsampling. The pooling layer reduces the dimensions of the data by combining outputs of a cluster of neurons at one layer into a single neuron in the next layer. The general pooling operators are max and average operations. Figure 5 shows a pooling layer. It serves to reduce the spatial size of features, amount of computation in the network, and number of parameters and also controls overfitting and improves adversarial robustness [60].

Fully Connected Layer

In a CNN, fully connected layers usually follow after several convolution and pooling layers. They will take high-level features generated by convolution or pooling layers and use them to classify input images. Neurons in a fully connected layer are fully connected to all the outputs of the previous layer, as seen in a regular feedforward neural network. The final output of fully connected layers is a vector of values, each representing the probability that a certain feature belongs to a class. Figure 6 shows a fully connected layer.

Recent CNN Architectures

As we have introduced types of layers used to build a CNN, we can now discuss how to design a CNN with these layers. One of the earliest CNN architectures was LeNet proposed by LeCun to automatically recognize handwritten zip code numbers [19, 20]. LeNet defines the basic components of CNN. Although LeNet achieved high performance, it was not widely adopted at that time due to the lack of powerful computers. Processing capacity limited the emergence of large-size CNNs, and LeNet architecture only contains 6 layers including 3 convolution layers, 2 pooling layers, and a fully connected layer.

Krizhevsky et al. [1] designed a CNN called AlexNet in 2012. AlexNet achieved an impressive top-5 error rate of 15.3% in the ImageNet LSVRC 2012 competition. Comparing to LeNet, AlexNet has 60-million parameters and 650,000 neurons and consists of 5 convolution layers, which are followed by 3 pooling layers and 3 fully connected layers [1]. It shows that the depth of a deep learning model is essential for its high performance. As AlexNet was trained on a large-scale dataset and has millions of parameters, it was computationally expensive. However, the training process can be performed efficiently due to the utilization of nonsaturating neurons and very efficient implementation of convolution operation with GPUs. AlexNet also contains many novel features to train networks faster and reduce overfitting, such as ReLU nonlinearity, local response normalization, and dropout.

AlexNet [1] shows that it was possible to train a deep CNN on large-scale datasets. Many new CNN architectures were proposed ever since. VGG was introduced by Simonyan and Zisserman [2], which included 16–19 lay-

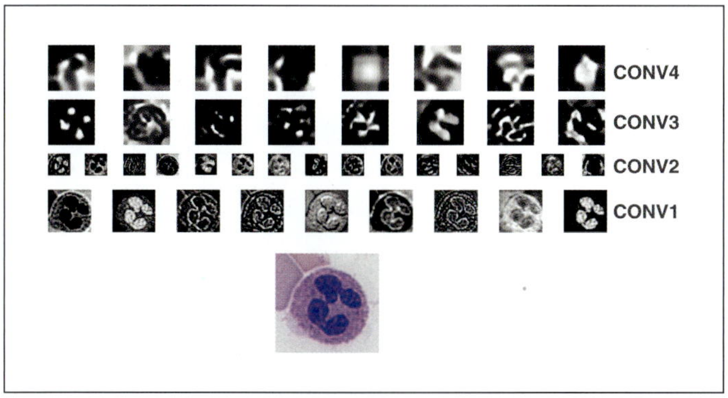

Fig. 8. Some feature maps of different convolution layers. The feature maps in convolution layers 3 and 4 have been magnified for easier observation.

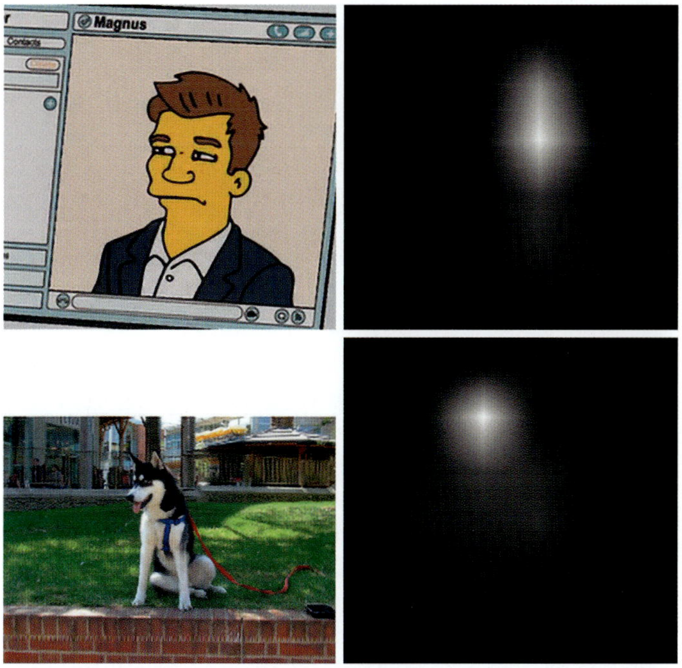

Fig. 9. The feature maps of 151st channel on the conv5 layer of a CNN model trained on ImageNet. It will be active on human and animal faces. CNN, convolution neural network.

ers. It has more efficient receptive fields due to the utilization of the stack of small convolution layers, which also makes it possible to design a deeper CNN for better performance.

As a CNN model goes deeper, it becomes more difficult to train due to the problem of vanishing or exploding gradients, which hampers convergence of the training process. The degradation problem was addressed by introducing a deep residual learning framework which is the essence of residual neural networks [3, 61]. The idea of a residual neural network is to reuse activations from a previous layer. A building block of the residual network is illustrated in Figure 7. A residual network is easier to optimize and can obtain high accuracy even with a very deep CNN. Comparing to 16-layer VGG, ResNet has developed 152-layer models on the ImageNet dataset and 1,000-layer models on the CIFAR10 dataset achieving high accuracy.

In recent years, many more CNN architectures were proposed such as GoogLeNet (Inception) and DenseNet [39, 62, 63] which not only include more layers but also have connections between various layers to strengthen feature propagation and reduce the number of parameters. A module of Inception is illustrated in Figure 7. Some small but powerful CNNs are used in mobile phones or computers without GPU. In mobile devices with limited power and processing capacity, lower performance is often acceptable to achieve better power efficiency. MobileNet, ShuffleNet [64], and EffNet [65] are several architectures running on mobile platforms.

With 3 types of layers, designing efficient architectures still requires a lot of expert knowledge and is a time-consuming and error-prone process. Hence, some researchers focus on NAS that is based on reinforcement learning [50, 66, 67] and gradient [68] or evolutionary methods [69, 70] to automatically generate good CNN architectures.

As we have gone through the major components of CNN architecture and deep learning, one issue particularly important to the medical field is how a deep learning model reaches certain decisions and whether the decision-making process is transparent and can be explained clearly. While interpretability and explainability of deep models are active in research, in the next section, we will try to illustrate some ideas through visualization.

Interpretability, Explainability, and Trustworthiness of Deep Learning Models

Although deep learning models have brought significant improvement in various medical imaging fields, how they work remains largely unknown. Even with recent works focusing on this important issue, there are still many open questions when it comes to explain and interpret deep learning models and their output [71–75]. In this section, we will introduce some insight into visualization techniques.

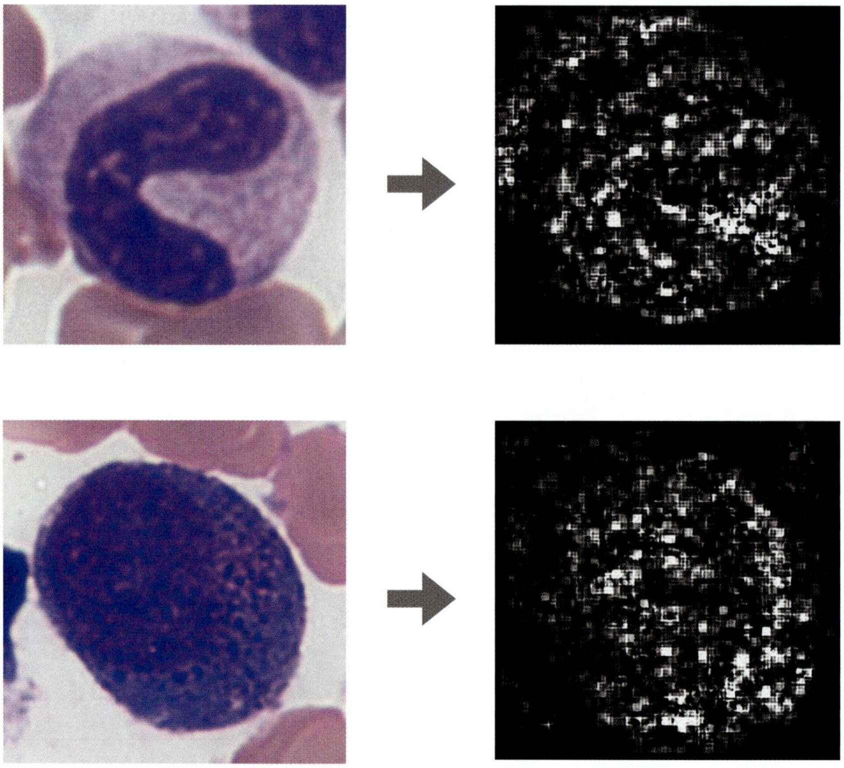

Fig. 10. Sensitivity map of bone marrow cells shows regions of input image that have significant influence on model predictions.

Feature Maps

Before CNNs are widely used in image processing, a general process of image recognition method includes preprocessing, feature extraction, and training a classifier based on extracted features [76]. Feature extraction is a crucial step to image recognition. The extracted features should contain distinguished information to recognize different classes and be insensitive to irrelevant noise in images. Feature extractors are usually designed based on various properties of images. For example, Haar-like features [77, 78] are commonly used in face recognition, histograms of oriented gradients [79], and deformable part models [80] that are often used in pedestrian detection. In some applications, such as medical images, expertise and domain-specific knowledge are required for designing feature extractors. For example, cell morphological information including the cell color, the shape of nucleus, the ratio of nucleus to cytoplasm, and cell texture [81–84] is a key feature to the classification of different types of nucleated cells found in peripheral blood and bone marrow. The extraction of morphological features requires professional knowledge of cytology.

Handcrafted features require careful tuning but offer interpretable results. However, the situation is different in CNNs. Although CNNs allow models to learn features automatically from images without feature engineering, the CNN along with many other machine learning models is often considered as a black box without knowing any of its internal workings. Hence, a key practical problem is what a CNN has learned. A straightforward method is to visualize feature maps that plot activation values for neurons in each layer of CNN in response to an image.

To illustrate this method, images of nucleated cells found in the bone marrow are used as an example to show some feature maps. The CNN model and image set used in this case are based on [85]. The illustrations of feature maps are shown in Figure 8. In these feature maps, we can see that some of them detect nucleus, some focus on cytoplasm, and so on. As layers of CNNs become higher, feature maps tend to represent more abstract higher-level features.

Yosinski et al. [86] noticed that some particular channels are found to respond to certain objects. For example, the 151st convolution filter on convolution layer 5 of a CNN trained on ImageNet responds to human and ani-

Acta Cytologica 2021;65:310–323
DOI: 10.1159/000510992

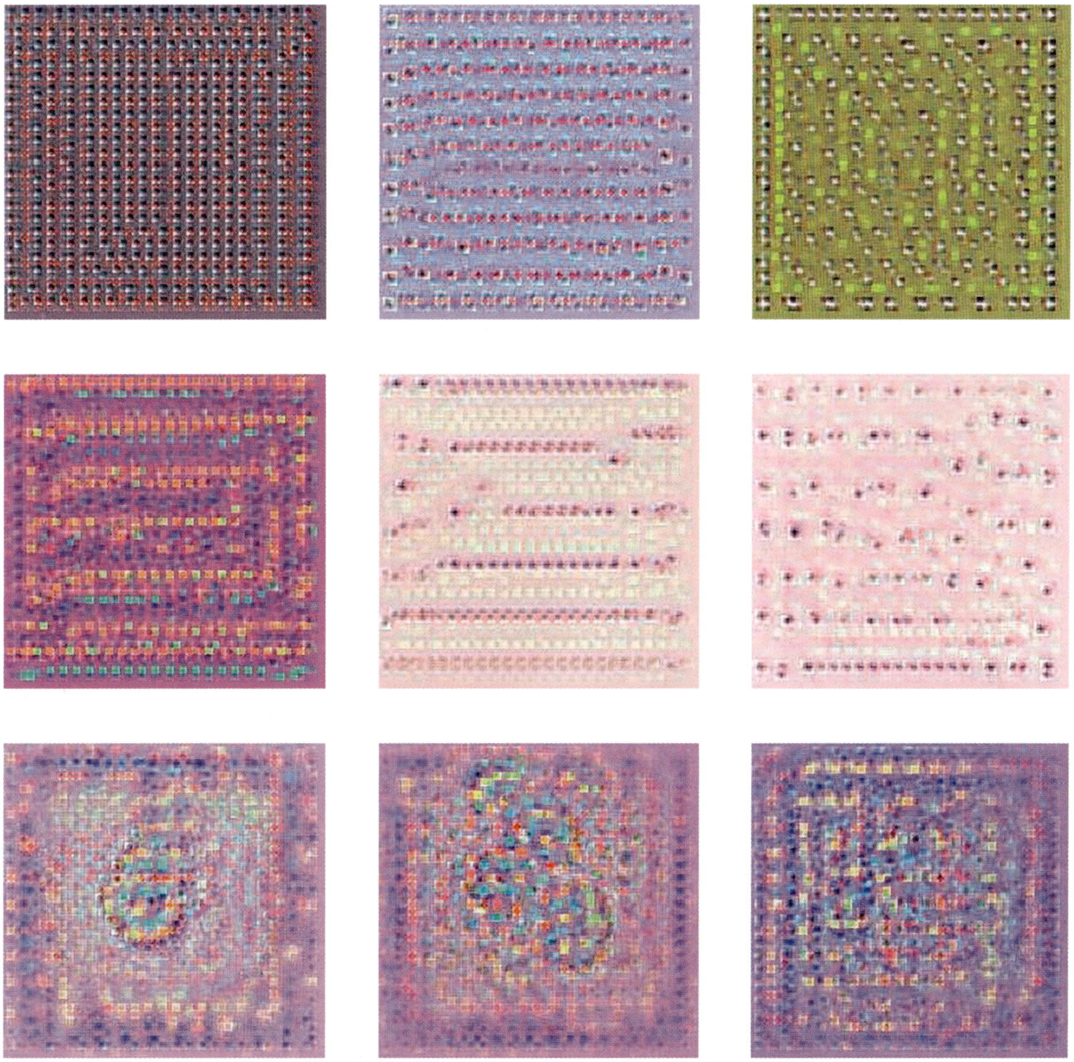

Fig. 11. Visualization of example features of convolution layer 1 (top row), convolution layer 2 (middle row), and fully connected layer (bottom row).

mal faces, as shown in Figure 9. It should be noted that the 151st convolution filter is not a single filter, but is a combination of multiple convolution filters. Unlike a small number of Haar-style filters utilized in face detection, CNNs usually have an enormous number of filters. Take the 151st convolution filter on conv5 of AlexNet as an example; it involves 270,624 filters. It is hard to understand how a CNN model works with so many filters.

Visualization Techniques for Better Interpretation

Instead of just visualizing the feature maps, there are some studies [28, 87–90] that try to find regions of an image that are influential to final classification results. Those methods are largely based on computing gradients of class score or specific convolution filters with respect to input images. Gradients of input images are regarded as sensitivity maps.

Sensitivity maps of CNNs reveal the region of input images that have significant influence on classification decisions. Sensitivity maps compute gradients of a model's prediction with respect to individual pixels, holding the weights fixed. As feature maps discussed in Section 4.1, the illustration of sensitivity maps based on the bone marrow cell dataset is shown in Figure 10.

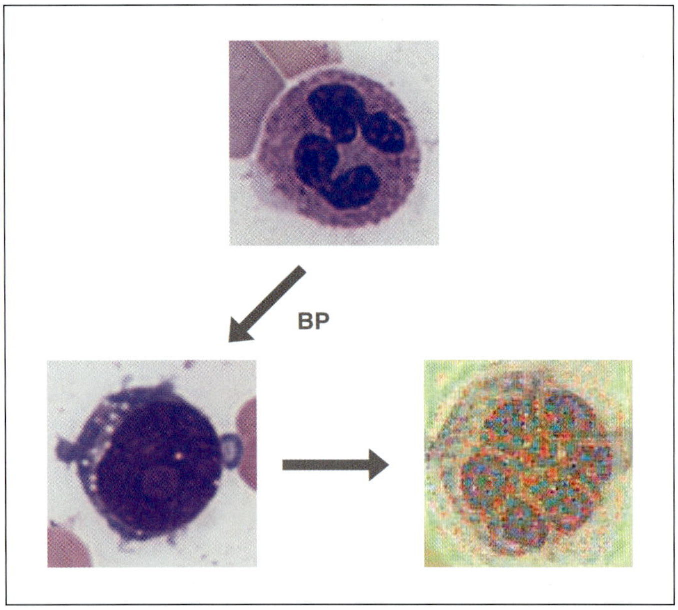

Fig. 12. To explore how the CNN recognizes neutrophils, we maximize the output of label neutrophil in a CNN whose input is lymphocyte. The nucleus of lymphocyte begins to become multilobed, which is the key characteristic of neutrophils. CNN, convolution neural network; BP, backpropagation.

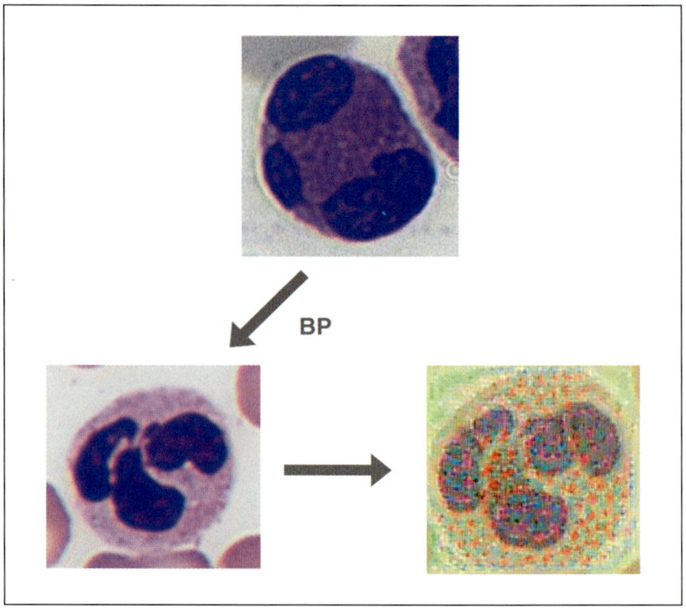

Fig. 13. To explore how the CNN recognizes eosinophils, we maximize the output of label eosinophil in a CNN whose input is neutrophil. The cytoplasm of neutrophils tends to be filled with large granules which is a discriminate feature of eosinophils. CNN, convolution neural network; BP, backpropagation.

Visualization of some specific convolution and connected layers is shown in Figure 11. This visualization is generated by maximizing the response of specific convolution filters or fully connected nodes through backpropagation while updating input and holding weights fixed. Images with random values assigned from a normal distribution are fed to a CNN model. After 50 iterations, we can compute preferred inputs for different channels on convolution or fully connected layers.

Instead of feeding images of normal distribution to the CNN, some randomly selected images from the bone marrow cell dataset are used to reveal the features that the CNN has learned. A lymphocyte image is input into the CNN; we try to maximize the output of label neutrophil by changing the input image. As shown in Figures 12 and 13, the nucleus of lymphocyte begins to become multilobed that is the key characteristic of neutrophils after 50 iterations. Similar results appear in neutrophils and eosinophils. Eosinophils have more and larger granules than neutrophils. Hence, if we use a neutrophil image as input and eosinophil as a target, the cytoplasm of neutrophil will be filled with large granules. These visualization methods show what features are learned by CNNs including some features consistent with the experience of medical experts such as multilobed nucleus in neutrophils and granules in eosinophils.

Discussion and Future Trends

Although the CNN has made significant progress in medical image processing, many challenges and open questions remain. The CNN is a data-driven approach like many other machine learning techniques. Training data used in the CNN require annotations, which are hindered by the cost and privacy constraints [91]. Medical data are highly imbalanced as the number of positive samples is usually much less than negative samples. Many methods have been proposed to address these challenges [92–94]. The CNN will continue to make progress in medical imaging. We think that 2 trends may have significant potential. First, multisource learning by integrating data from heterogeneous data sources may improve model performance when only a limited amount of medical data are available. For example, when examining the bone marrow, a doctor usually not only relies on microscope images but also considers clinical information and other test results for better diagnosis. Second, to save high annotation cost, unsupervised learning has significant potential in the medical imaging field to find hidden patterns in unlabeled data with minimum human involvement [95].

Statement of Ethics

No human subjects were involved in this survey study.

Conflict of Interest Statement

The authors have no conflicts of interest to declare.

Funding Sources

None of the authors received any funding for this study.

Author Contributions

Z.H. and P.C. contributed to the writing of this paper. Q.L. and J.L. contributed to the paper structure and revision. J.F. and J.H. contributed to the data collection, figure preparation, and writing of this paper.

References

1 Krizhevsky A, Sutskever I, Hinton GE. ImageNet classification with deep convolution neural networks. In: Pereira F, Burges CJC, Bottou L, Weinberger KQ, editors. Advances in neural information processing systems 25; 2012. p. 1097–105.

2 Simonyan K, Zisserman A. Very deep convolution networks for large scale image recognition. In: International conference on learning representations; 2015.

3 He K, Zhang X, Ren S, Sun J. Deep residual learning for image recognition. The IEEE conference on computer vision and pattern recognition (CVPR); 2016.

4 McCarthy J, Minsky ML, Rochester N, Shannon CE. A proposal for the Dartmouth summer research project on artificial intelligence, August 31, 1955. AI Mag. 2006;27(4):12.

5 Deng J, Dong W, Socher R, Li LJ, Li K, Fei-Fei L. ImageNet: a large scale hierarchical image database. 2009 IEEE conference on computer vision and pattern recognition. IEEE; 2009. p. 248–55.

6 Hinton GE, Osindero S, Teh YW. A fast learning algorithm for deep belief nets. Neural Comput. 2006;18(7):1527–54.

7 Hinton G. Deep belief networks. Scholarpedia. 2009;4(5):5947.

8 LeCun Y, Bengio Y, Hinton G. Deep learning. Nature. 2015;521(7553):436–44.

9 Schuster M, Paliwal KK. Bidirectional recurrent neural networks. IEEE Trans Signal Process. 1997;45(11):2673–81.

10 Hou L, Samaras D, Kurc TM, Gao Y, Davis JE, Saltz JH. Patch-based convolution neural network for whole slide tissue image classification. In: Proceedings of the IEEE conference on computer vision and pattern recognition; 2016. p. 2424–33.

11 Rajpurkar P, Irvin J, Zhu K, Yang B, Mehta H, Duan T, et al. CheXNet: radiologist-level pneumonia detection on chest X-rays with deep learning. arXiv preprint arXiv:171105225. 2017.

12 Gulshan V, Peng L, Coram M, Stumpe MC, Wu D, Narayanaswamy A, et al. Development and validation of a deep learning algorithm for detection of diabetic retinopathy in retinal fundus photographs. JAMA. 2016;316(22): 2402–10.

13 Girshick R, Donahue J, Darrell T, Malik J. Rich feature hierarchies for accurate object detection and semantic segmentation. In: Proceedings of the IEEE Conference on Computer Vision and Pattern Recognition; 2014. p. 580–87.

14 He K, Gkioxari G, Dollár P, Girshick R. Mask r-cnn. In: Proceedings of the IEEE International Conference on Computer Vision; 2017. p. 2961–69.

15 Collobert R, Weston J, Bottou L, Karlen M, Kavukcuoglu K, Kuksa P. Natural language processing (almost) from scratch. J Mach Learn Res. 2011;12(Aug):2493–537.

16 Manning CD, Surdeanu M, Bauer J, Finkel JR, Bethard S, McClosky D. The Stanford CoreNLP natural language processing toolkit. In: Proceed-ings of 52nd annual meeting of the association for computational linguistics: system demonstrations; 2014. p. 55–60.

17 Fukushima K. Neocognitron: a self-organizing neural network model for a mechanism of pattern recognition unaffected by shift in position. Biol Cybern. 1980;36(4):193–202.

18 Fukushima K. Analysis of the process of visual pattern recognition by the neocognitron. Neural Networks. 1989;2(6):413–20.

19 LeCun Y, Boser B, Denker JS, Henderson D, Howard RE, Hubbard W, et al. Backpropagation applied to handwritten zip code recognition. Nat Commun. 1989;1(4):541–51.

20 LeCun Y, Bottou L, Bengio Y, Haffner P. Gradient-based learning applied to document recognition. Proc IEEE. 1998;86(11):2278–324.

21 Girshick R. Fast r-cnn. In: Proceedings of the IEEE International Conference on Computer Vision; 2015. p. 1440–48.

22 Redmon J, Divvala S, Girshick R, Farhadi A. You only look once: unified, real-time object detection. In: Proceedings of the IEEE Conference on Computer Vision and Pattern Recognition; 2016. p. 779–88.

23 Liu W, Anguelov D, Erhan D, Szegedy C, Reed S, Fu CY, et al. Ssd: single shot multibox detector. European Conference on Computer Vision. Springer; 2016. p. 21–37.

24 Chen LC, Papandreou G, Kokkinos I, Murphy K, Yuille AL. DeepLab: semantic image segmentation with deep convolution nets, atrous convolution, and fully connected CRFS. IEEE Trans Pattern Anal Mach Intel. 2017;40(4):834–48.

25 Badrinarayanan V, Kendall A, Cipolla R. SegNet: a deep convolution encoder decoder architecture for image segmentation. IEEE Trans Pattern Anal Mach Intel. 2017;39(12): 2481–95.

26 Cordts M, Omran M, Ramos S, Rehfeld T, Enzweiler M, Benenson R, et al. The cityscapes dataset for semantic urban scene understanding. In: Proceedings of the IEEE conference on computer vision and pattern recognition; 2016, p. 3213–23.

27 Lin G, Milan A, Shen C, Reid I. RefineNet: multi-path refinement networks for high-resolution semantic segmentation. In: Proceedings of the IEEE Conference on Computer Vision and Pattern Recognition; 2017. p. 1925–34.

28 Simonyan K, Vedaldi A, Zisserman A. Deep inside convolution networks: visualising image classification models and saliency maps. arXiv preprint arXiv:13126034. 2013.

29 Xie Y, Kong X, Xing F, Liu F, Su H, Yang L. Deep voting: a robust approach toward nucleus localization in microscopy images. International conference on medical image computing and computer-ssisted Intervention. Springer; 2015. p. 374–82.

30 Sanyal P, Mukherjee T, Barui S, Das A, Gangopadhyay P. Artificial intelligence in cytopathology: a neural network to identify papillary carcinoma on thyroid fine-needle aspiration cytology smears. J Pathol Inform. 2018;9:43.

31 Sanghvi AB, Allen EZ, Callenberg KM, Pantanowitz L. Performance of an artificial intelligence algorithm for reporting urine cytopathology. Cancer Cytopathol. 2019 Oct; 127(10):658–66.

32 Sadanandan SK, Ranefall P, Le Guyader S, Wählby C. Automated training of deep convolutional neural networks for cell segmentation. Sci Rep. 2017;7(1):7860–7.

33 Liang Z, Powell A, Ersoy I, Poostchi M, Silamut K, Palaniappan K, et al. CNN-based image analysis for malaria diagnosis. In: 2016 IEEE international conference on bioinformatics and biomedicine (BIBM). IEEE; 2016 Dec 15. p. 493–6.
34 Li X, Li W, Xu X, Hu W. Cell classification using convolutional neural networks in medical hyperspectral imagery. In: 2017 2nd international conference on image, vision and computing (ICIVC). IEEE; 2017 Jun 2. p. 501–4.
35 Ciresan DC, Giusti A, Gambardella LM, Schmidhuber J. Mitosis detection in breast cancer histology images with deep neural networks. International conference on medical image computing and computer-assisted intervention. Springer; 2013. p. 411–8.
36 Araújo T, Aresta G, Castro E, Rouco J, Aguiar P, Eloy C, et al. Classification of breast cancer histology images using convolutional neural networks. PLoS One. 2017;12(6):e0177544.
37 Bardou D, Zhang K, Ahmad SM. Classification of breast cancer based on histology images using convolutional neural networks. IEEE Access. 2018;6:24680–93.
38 Li Y, Ping W. Cancer metastasis detection with neural conditional random field. arXiv preprint arXiv: 180607064. 2018.
39 Szegedy C, Vanhoucke V, Ioffe S, Shlens J, Wojna Z. Rethinking the inception architecture for computer vision. In: Proceedings of the IEEE conference on computer vision and pattern recognition; 2016. p. 2818–26.
40 Zeng X, Chen H, Luo Y, Ye W. Automated diabetic retinopathy detection based on binocular Siamese-like convolutional neural network. IEEE Access. 2019;7:30744–53.
41 Wang X, Peng Y, Lu L, Lu Z, Bagheri M, Summers RM. ChestX-ray8: hospital scale chest X-ray database and benchmarks on weakly supervised classification and localization of common thorax diseases. In: Proceedings of the IEEE Conference on Computer Vision and Pattern Recognition; 2017. p. 2097–106.
42 Zhou B, Khosla A, Lapedriza A, Oliva A, Torralba A. Learning deep features for discriminative localization. In: Proceedings of the IEEE Conference on Computer Vision and Pattern Recognition; 2016. p. 2921–29.
43 Li L, Qin L, Xu Z, Yin Y, Wang X, Kong B, et al. Artificial intelligence distinguishes COVID-19 from community acquired pneumonia on chest CT. Radiology. 2020:200905.
44 Wang L, Wong A. COVID-Net: a tailored deep convolution neural network design for detection of COVID-19 cases from chest radiography images. arXiv preprint arXiv:200309871. 2020.
45 Apostolopoulos ID, Mpesiana TA. Covid-19: automatic detection from X-ray images utilizing transfer learning with convolution neural networks. Phys Eng Sci Med. 2020;43(2):635–40.
46 Ciresan D, Giusti A, Gambardella LM, Schmidhuber J. Deep neural networks segment neuronal membranes in electron microscopy images. Adv Neural Inf Process Syst. 2012;843–51.
47 Ronneberger O, Fischer P, Brox T. U-Net: convolution networks for biomedical image segmentation. In: International Conference on Medical Image Computing and Computer-Assisted Intervention. Springer; 2015. p. 234–41.
48 Milletari F, Navab N, Ahmadi SA. V-Net: fully convolution neural networks for volumetric medical image segmentation. In: 2016 Fourth International Conference on 3D Vision (3DV). IEEE; 2016. p. 565–71.
49 Kamnitsas K, Ledig C, Newcombe VF, Simpson JP, Kane AD, Menon DK, et al. Efficient multi-scale 3D CNN with fully connected CRF for accurate brain lesion segmentation. Med Image Anal. 2017;36:61–78.
50 Zoph B, Le QV. Neural architecture search with reinforcement learning. arXiv preprint arXiv:161101578. 2016.
51 Liu C, Chen LC, Schroff F, Adam H, Hua W, Yuille AL, et al. Auto-deeplab: Hierarchical neural architecture search for semantic image segmentation. In: Proceedings of the IEEE Conference on Computer Vision and Pattern Recognition; 2019. p. 82–92.
52 Hecht-Nielsen R. Theory of the backpropagation neural network. Neural networks for perception. Elsevier; 1992. p. 65–93.
53 Rumelhart DE, Hinton GE, Williams RJ. Learning internal representations by error propagation. California Univ San Diego La Jolla Inst for Cognitive Science; 1985.
54 Rumelhart DE, Durbin R, Golden R, Chauvin Y. Backpropagation: the basic theory. Backpropagation: theory, architectures and applications. 1995. p. 1–34.
55 Lowe DG. Distinctive image features from scale-invariant keypoints. Int J Comput Vis. 2004 Nov;60(2):91–110.
56 Lazebnik S, Schmid C, Ponce J. Beyond bags of features: spatial pyramid matching for recognizing natural scene categories. In: 2006 IEEE Computer Society Conference on Computer Vision and Pattern Recognition (CVPR'06); 2006. Vol. 2; p. 2169–78.
57 Le H, Borji A. What are the receptive, effective receptive, and projective fields of neurons in convolution neural networks? arXiv preprint arXiv:170507049. 2017.
58 Ghrare SE, Mohd. Ali MA, Jumari K, Ismail M. An efficient low complexity lossless coding algorithm for medical images. Am J App Sci. 2009;6(8):1502–8.
59 Kil SK, Lee JS, Shen DF, Ryu J, Lee EH, Min HK, et al. Lossless medical image compression using redundancy analysis. 2006.
60 Xie C, Wu Y, Maaten Lvd, Yuille AL, He K. Feature denoising for improving adversarial robustness. In: Proceedings of the IEEE Conference on Computer Vision and Pattern Recognition; 2019. p. 501–9.
61 Xie S, Girshick R, Dollár P, Tu Z, He K. Aggregated residual transformations for deep neural networks. In: Proceedings of the IEEE Conference on Computer Vision and Pattern Recognition; 2017. p. 1492–1500.
62 Szegedy C, Liu W, Jia Y, Sermanet P, Reed S, Anguelov D, et al. Going deeper with convolutions. In: Proceedings of the IEEE Conference on Computer Vision and Pattern Recognition; 2015. p. 1–9.
63 Szegedy C, Ioffe S, Vanhoucke V, Alemi AA. Inception-v4, Inception-ResNet and the impact of residual connections on learning. In: Thirty-First AAAI Conference on Artificial Intelligence; 2017.
64 Ma N, Zhang X, Zheng HT, Sun J. ShuffleNet v2: Practical guidelines for efficient cnn architecture design. In: Proceedings of the European Conference on Computer Vision (ECCV); 2018. p. 116–31.
65 Freeman I, Roese Koerner L, Kummert A. EffNet: an efficient structure for convolution neural networks. In: 2018 25th IEEE International Conference on Image Processing (ICIP). IEEE; 2018. p. 6–10.
66 Zoph B, Vasudevan V, Shlens J, Le QV. Learning transferable architectures for scalable image recognition. In: Proceedings of the IEEE Conference on Computer Vision and Pattern Recognition; 2018. p. 8697–710.
67 Zhong Z, Yan J, Liu CL. Practical network blocks design with q-learning. arXiv preprint arXiv:170805552. 2017. p. 6.
68 Liu H, Simonyan K, Yang Y. Darts: differentiable architecture search. arXiv preprint arXiv:180609055. 2018.
69 Real E, Moore S, Selle A, Saxena S, Suematsu YL, Tan J, et al. Large scale evolution of image classifiers. In: Proceedings of the 34th International Conference on Machine Learning-Volume 70. JMLR.org; 2017. p. 2902–11.
70 Xie L, Yuille A. Genetic cnn. In: Proceedings of the IEEE International Conference on Computer Vision; 2017. p. 1379–88.
71 Haeffele BD, Vidal R. Global optimality in neural network training. In: Proceedings of the IEEE Conference on Computer Vision and Pattern Recognition; 2017. p. 7331–39.
72 Shwartz-Ziv R, Tishby N. Opening the black box of deep neural networks via information. arXiv preprint arXiv:170300810. 2017.
73 Kuo CCJ. Understanding convolutional neural networks with a mathematical model. J Vis Commun Image R. 2016;41:406–13.
74 Baral C, Fuentes O, Kreinovich V. Why deep neural networks: a possible theoretical explanation. Constraint programming and decision making: theory and applications. Springer; 2018. p. 1–5.
75 Saxe AM, Bansal Y, Dapello J, Advani M, Kolchinsky A, Tracey BD, et al. On the information bottleneck theory of deep learning. J Stat Mech. 2019;2019(12):124020.

76 Everingham M, Van Gool L, Williams CKI, Winn J, Zisserman A. The Pascal visual object classes (voc) challenge. Int J Comput Vis. 2010;88(2):303–38.
77 Viola P, Jones M. Rapid object detection using a boosted cascade of simple features. In: Proceedings of the 2001 IEEE Computer Society Conference on Computer Vision and Pattern Recognition. CVPR 2001. IEEE; 2001. Vol. 1; p. I.
78 Lienhart R, Maydt J. An extended set of haar-like features for rapid object detection. In: Proceedings International Conference on Image Processing. IEEE; 2002. Vol. 1. p. I.
79 Dalal N, Triggs B. Histograms of oriented gradients for human detection. In: 2005 IEEE Computer Society Conference on Computer Vision and Pattern Recognition (CVPR'05); 2005. Vol. 1; p. 886–93.
80 Felzenszwalb PF, Girshick RB, McAllester D. Cascade object detection with deformable part models. In: 2010 IEEE Computer Society Conference on Computer Vision and Pattern Recognition. IEEE; 2010. p. 2241–8.
81 Scotti F. Automatic morphological analysis for acute leukemia identification in peripheral blood microscope images. In: CIMSA. 2005 IEEE International Conference on Computational Intelligence for Measurement Systems and Applications, 2005. IEEE; 2005. p. 96–101.
82 Rezatofighi SH, Soltanian-Zadeh H. Automatic recognition of five types of white blood cells in peripheral blood. Comput Med Imaging Graph. 2011;35(4):333–43.
83 Theera-Umpon N, Dhompongsa S. Morphological granulometric features of nucleus in automatic bone marrow white blood cell classification. IEEE Trans Inf Technol Biomed. 2007;11(3):353–9.
84 Theera-Umpon N. White blood cell segmentation and classification in microscopic bone marrow images. In: International Conference on Fuzzy Systems and Knowledge Discovery. Springer; 2005. p. 787–96.
85 Chen M, Xu X, Zhang J, Peng X, Tang G, Fengqi F, et al. Automatic bone marrow cell classification on digital images by an artificial intelligence (AI)-based system: a pilot study. In: Laboratory investigation. New York, NY: Nature Publishing Group; 2019. Vol. 99.
86 Yosinski J, Clune J, Nguyen A, Fuchs T, Lipson H. Understanding neural networks through deep visualization. arXiv preprint arXiv:150606579. 2015.
87 Zeiler MD, Fergus R. Visualizing and understanding convolution networks. European Conference on Computer Vision. Springer; 2014. p. 818–33.
88 Shrikumar A, Greenside P, Kundaje A. Learning important features through propagating activation differences. In: Proceedings of the 34th International Conference on Machine Learning. JMLR.org; 2017. Vol. 70; p. 3145–53.
89 Smilkov D, Thorat N, Kim B, Viégas F, Wattenberg M. SmoothGrad: removing noise by adding noise. arXiv preprint arXiv:170603825. 2017.
90 Adebayo J, Gilmer J, Muelly M, Goodfellow I, Hardt M, Kim B. Sanity checks for saliency maps. Adv Neural Inf Process Syst; 2018. p. 9505–15.
91 Greenspan H, Van Ginneken B, Summers RM. Guest editorial deep learning in medical imaging: overview and future promise of an exciting new technique. IEEE Trans Med Imaging. 2016;35(5):1153–9.
92 Buda M, Maki A, Mazurowski MA. A systematic study of the class imbalance problem in convolutional neural networks. Neural Netw. 2018;106:249–59.
93 Johnson JM, Khoshgoftaar TM. Survey on deep learning with class imbalance. J Big Data. 2019;6(1):27.
94 Guan MY, Gulshan V, Dai AM, Hinton GE. Who said what: modeling individual labelers improves classification. In: Thirty-Second AAAI Conference on Artificial Intelligence; 2018.
95 Barlow HB. Unsupervised learning. Neural Comput. 1989;1(3):295–311.

Acta Cytologica

Review

Acta Cytologica 2021;65:324–329
DOI: 10.1159/000512097

Received: June 18, 2020
Accepted: October 6, 2020
Published online: December 16, 2020

Artificial Intelligence in Thyroid Fine Needle Aspiration Biopsies

Brie Kezlarian Oscar Lin

Department of Pathology, Memorial Sloan Kettering Cancer Center, New York, NY, USA

Keywords
Artificial intelligence · Machine learning · Thyroid fine needle aspiration biopsy

Abstract
Background: From cell phones to aerospace, artificial intelligence (AI) has wide-reaching influence in the modern age. In this review, we discuss the application of AI solutions to an equally ubiquitous problem in cytopathology – thyroid fine needle aspiration biopsy (FNAB). Thyroid nodules are common in the general population, and FNAB is the sampling modality of choice. The resulting prevalence in the practicing pathologist's daily workload makes thyroid FNAB an appealing target for the application of AI solutions. ***Summary:*** This review summarizes all available literature on the application of AI to thyroid cytopathology. We follow the evolution from morphometric analysis to convolutional neural networks. We explore the application of AI technology to different questions in thyroid cytopathology, including distinguishing papillary carcinoma from benign, distinguishing follicular adenoma from carcinoma and identifying non-invasive follicular thyroid neoplasm with papillary-like nuclear features by key words and phrases. ***Key Messages:*** The current literature shows promise towards the application of AI technology to thyroid fine needle aspiration biopsy. Much work is needed to define how this powerful technology will be of best use to the future of cytopathology practice.

Introduction

Pathology is at the dawn of a major paradigm shift with increased applications of digital and computational pathology. The standard practice of using a light microscope for diagnosis has remained largely unchanged for over a century. This diagnostic model has been transforming since the advent of digital pathology. Glass slides are being digitized into whole slide images (WSIs) more frequently, a process facilitated by the introduction of high-output digital slide scanners. The digital images created from WSIs have allowed the development of the field of computational pathology which uses the massive amount of data generated to facilitate computer-assisted diagnostics [1, 2]. Recent advances in deep learning [3] in solving image classification tasks, such as classification and categorization, have revolutionized the field. Some high-capacity deep neural network models have been reported to be comparable to human performance [4]. Although most current efforts have centered on the evaluation of histologic sections, it is important to remember that one of the earliest commercial applications of computational pathology was a cytology-centered application for cervico-vaginal cytology specimens (Papnet). Although not commercially successful, many other investigators have evaluated the use of computational pathology tools such as artificial intelligence (AI) in different types of cytology specimens. Among the different types of cytology specimens evaluated, thyroid fine needle aspira-

Oscar Lin
Department of Pathology, Memorial Sloan-Kettering Cancer Center
1275 York Avenue
New York NY 10065 (USA)
lino@mskcc.org

tion biopsy (FNAB) cytology specimens are of particular interest due to their potential clinical impact. Thyroid nodules are reported to occur in 19–68% of randomly selected individuals, with higher frequencies in women and the elderly [5, 6], and this incidence has dramatically increased with the advent of high-resolution ultrasound. The main clinical issue is the need to rule out thyroid cancer in all these thyroid nodules, which occurs in 7–15% of cases depending on age, sex, radiation exposure history, family history, and other factors [7]. To address this issue, FNAB of these thyroid nodules is recommended according to their size and radiological appearance [8].

The sensitivity and specificity of thyroid FNAB are reported to be 68–98% and 56–100%, respectively. However, 15–30% of thyroid FNAB are classified as indeterminate. Approximately 25% of the indeterminate cases will be diagnosed as malignant in surgical resections, suggesting that a large proportion of surgeries are unnecessary [9–12]. Although tests based on molecular profiling of thyroid FNAB have been developed in an attempt to refine the diagnosis among indeterminate thyroid FNAB diagnosis, these molecular tests show limitations and demonstrate variable sensitivity and specificity among the several commercially available tests [13, 14]. AI, including machine learning, has the hypothetical capability to further refine the evaluation of thyroid FNAB specimens. Several investigators have studied the use of AI in thyroid FNAB, and their work is summarized below.

Early Studies: Benign versus Malignant

The literature on AI solutions in thyroid cytopathology predates the recent AI boom by over a decade [15]. In 1996, Karakitsos et al. [16] attempted to classify benign and malignant follicular and Hurtle cell lesions using a neural network. Geometric and densometric features of approximately 100 nuclei from each of the 51 patients' Giemsa-stained smears were measured. Using these measurements, 2 different neural networks were trained and tested. The first attempted to classify the cell into one of the 4 categories: benign follicular cell, benign oncocyte, malignant follicular cell, and malignant oncocyte. This performed reasonably well on the training set data (82.24, 76.28, 95.12, and 68.19% of cells correctly classified for follicular cells, benign oncocytes, malignant follicular cells [i.e., papillary carcinoma], and malignant oncocytes, respectively). The test data were less impressive (47.97, 57.25, 71.32, and 26.86% of cells correctly classified for follicular cells, benign oncocytes, malignant follicular cells, and malignant oncocytes, respectively). The second classifier simply attempted to categorize the nucleus as benign or malignant. This performed much better than the four-class classifier at test time, achieving 91.12 and 89.64% for benign and malignant nuclei, respectively, correctly classified for an overall accuracy of 90.61% on test data.

This same group performed a similar study using a learning vector quantizer neural network [16]. This time, the vectorized input were the mean and standard deviations of the measured morphometric data per case. The four-class classifier results were not impressive. The authors postulated that the classifier had difficulty distinguishing oncocytic from follicular lesions. The two-class classifier was able to distinguish benign from malignant lesions with 94.9% sensitivity and 98.9% specificity.

Later studies by this group abandoned the four-class classifier and focused on distinguishing benign from malignant lesions. In their study published in 2006 [17], the authors used morphometric nuclear data extrapolated from May Grunwald-Giemsa-stained smears. Nuclei were categorized into either benign or malignant using 4 independent classifiers: a linear classifier, a two-layer feed-forward neural network, 3 two-layer feed-forward networks combined by the Adaboost algorithm, and a K-nearest neighbour classifier. If the percentage of benign nuclei in a given case exceeded the average between the maximum percentage of nuclei called benign by the classifier in a malignant case and the minimum percentage of nuclei called benign in a benign case, that case was classified as benign. The most successful classifier on test data was the combination of 3 two-layer feed-forward networks generated by the Adaboost algorithm with 5 nodes, though notably this only outperformed the K-nearest neighbour classifier by 0.56%.

Gopinath et al. [18–20] published several studies with a similar approach to classify thyroid tumours into benign versus malignant lesions. In this case, statistical textural features from images of thyroid lesions were input into one or more classifiers, including decision tree, K-nearest neighbour, Elman neural network, and support vector machine. These studies were problematic, however, as the input data were images taken from the Papanicolaou Society of Cytopathology online atlas. Because the classifier was trained by and tested on textbook images, it is unlikely that the results would be widely applicable to real-world applications. This is one example of overfitting. Overfitting occurs when the AI's concept for what constitutes ground truth is too narrow. The issue of overfitting most commonly arises in the context of small sample size or when the training data have insufficient variation to capture the variation seen in practice.

Acta Cytologica 2021;65:324–329
DOI: 10.1159/000512097

Convolutional Neural Networks to Determine Benign from Malignant

More recent studies utilize convolutional neural networks (CNNs) for analysis. CNNs are ideal for image analysis because unlike other neural network architectures, CNNs retain spatial information while moving from one layer to the next. Few papers have been written applying CNNs to thyroid cytopathology. All narrowed their focus to distinguishing papillary thyroid carcinomas (PTCs) from non-PTCs.

Sanyal et al. [21] published on CNNs to assess thyroid nodules in 2018. They trained their algorithm on 186 images of PTCs and 184 images of goitre, lymphocytic thyroiditis, and nodules cytologically diagnosed as follicular lesions. These images were taken from Romanowsky-stained smears at ×10 and ×40 objective magnifications and then cropped to 512 × 512 pixel images. The evaluation dataset comprised 174 images taken from 10 different smears. The same 21 foci of PTCs and 66 foci of non-PTCs were photographed at both ×10 and ×40 objective magnifications. The images were analyzed separately, and then the data for each focus were compiled. When either the ×10 or the ×40 objective magnification images were required to be called positive to consider the lesion malignant, the algorithm demonstrated a sensitivity and specificity of 90.48 and 83.33%, respectively. If both the ×10 and the ×40 objective magnification images were required to classify a lesion as malignant, the sensitivity (33.33%) suffered significantly at the hands of an admittedly impressive increase in specificity (98.48%).

Guan et al. [22] subsequently published on the use of a CNN experiment using 224 × 224 pixel images of liquid-based preparations (Surepath stained with hematoxylin and eosin) taken at ×40 objective magnifications. Two separate AI architectures, VGG-16 [23] and Inception-v3 [24], were trained on 407 images of PTCs and 352 images of benign nodules and then tested on 69 PTC images and 59 images of benign nodules. All 887 images were taken from 20 Surepath slides and the images randomly assigned into the test and training sets. In an ideal scenario, the test and training cases would be completely separate. The data showed the VGG-16 model was able to predict the correct category with 100% sensitivity and 94.91% specificity. The Inception-v3 model achieved a sensitivity of 98.55%, with a specificity of 86.44%, though it is difficult to ascertain the influence training and testing different images of the same tumour had on the results.

These studies represent a significant step forward as the first use of CNNs to investigate FNAB of thyroid nodules. In distinction from previous studies, the authors use images rather than data extracted from images as input. However, the methodology still requires a significant amount of hands-on preprocessing. Elliott Range et al. [25] published the first paper to use WSIs as input to a CNN architecture without hands-on preprocessing steps. They utilized a semi-supervised method comprised of 2 CNNs. The first identified regions of interest, using pathologist-annotated areas containing follicular cells as ground truth. The second CNN classified these regions of interest into benign or malignant categories, using the surgical resection diagnosis as ground truth. Both CNNs were predicated on the VGG-11 [23] framework. This training methodology produced an algorithm that was able to predict a benign or malignant outcome with 92.0% sensitivity and 90.5% specificity.

They also developed cutoffs to approximate the Bethesda System for Reporting Thyroid Cytopathology (TBSRTC) category for each case using an ordinal regression framework. TBSRTC is not a strictly ordinal system, so these categories are not completely analogous, but the results were interesting nonetheless. In the test set comprised of 109 cases, 29 were called benign, with an associated risk of malignancy (ROM) of 0% and 10 were called malignant with a ROM of 100%. Concerning the less definitive categories, 48 were categorized atypia of undetermined significance with a ROM of 4.2%, 14 were identified as follicular nodules with a ROM of 50%, and 8 were called suspicious, with a ROM of 75%.

Non-Graphical Input to Determine Benign from Malignant

While image analysis seems like the most obvious application of AI technology to the analysis of thyroid, several groups have taken a different approach. Instead, Zoulias et al. [26] reviewed 1,886 non-malignant and 150 malignant smears notating the presence or absence of 67 microscopic features. These data were used to train an artificial neural network, support vector machine, and K-nearest neighbour [26]. These were both analyzed separately and using a majority voting classifier. The majority voting classifier, which combined the results of all 3 algorithms, outperformed each algorithm separately, with a sensitivity of 89.1% and a specificity of 99.4%.

Similarly, Ippolito et al. [27] used pathologist-defined microscopic characteristics but also integrated clinical data and ultrasound characteristics into their algorithm. Their aim was to triage indeterminate and follicular lesions into high- or low-risk categories using a neural network framework. Their algorithm demonstrated a sensitivity of 85.7% and a specificity of 58.8%.

Follicular Adenoma versus Carcinoma

The distinction between follicular adenoma and follicular carcinoma currently requires a surgical resection to evaluate for capsular and vascular invasion. Determination of benign from malignant follicular lesions by FNAB is a problem for which a solution continues to evade cytopathologists. This is exactly the problem for which Shapiro et al. [28] and Savala et al. [29] sought an AI solution. Shapiro et al. [28] trained 3 two-layer automated neural networks on different sets of data. The first was trained on pathologist-identified cytologic features, including the presence of colloid, structure of the tissue fragments, and cytoplasmic and nuclear features. The second used morphometric features as input data. The third neural network used 256 × 256 pixel colour images of Giemsa-stained smears. The cytologic, morphometric, and image algorithms correctly classified 93, 96, and 87% of cases, respectively.

Savala et al. [29] also sought an AI solution to delineate follicular adenoma from follicular carcinoma. The neural network architecture they employed was slightly deeper with 5 hidden nodes. They used a combination of both semiquantitatively evaluated cytologic features and morphometric parameters. The sample size was relatively small, with 26 cases of follicular adenoma and 31 cases of follicular carcinoma in total. The algorithm was able to correctly categorize the 3 follicular adenomas and 6 follicular carcinomas in the testing set.

Non-Invasive Follicular Thyroid Neoplasm with Papillary-Like Nuclear Features versus Papillary Carcinoma

Non-invasive follicular thyroid neoplasm with papillary-like nuclear features (NIFTP) is a low-risk neoplasm [30] that might not require surgical treatment. As a result, the distinction between NIFTP and PTC is clinically essential. Similar to follicular adenoma and carcinoma, a resection specimen is currently required to make this distinction in order to fully evaluate for presence of papillary formations and invasion. Maleki and colleagues [31] used a novel approach to the application of AI technologies to this important question. They processed key words and phrases from the microscopic descriptions, which were then used to train a support vector machine. There was not a separate test cohort, but the validation showed a sensitivity of 72.6% and a specificity of 81.6%.

Perhaps, the most interesting outcome of this study was the generation of weights for the key words and phrases. The weights reflected how often each key word or phrase was associated with a given outcome (i.e., NIFTP or PTC). The top 2 key words/phrases in favour of NIFTP over classic PTC were "scant colloid" and "microfollicular pattern." The top 2 words/phrases in favour of cPTC were "papillary" and "pale chromatin." While more study is needed, this novel approach could be applied to the generation of diagnostic criteria in the future.

Practical Applications

These studies represent over 2 decades of research applying a variety of AI technologies to evaluate thyroid cytology specimens. Unfortunately, no application has demonstrated to be robust enough for clinical use. Currently, there are still significant technologic hurdles that must be addressed before AI applications to thyroid FNAB are ready for clinical use.

One issue is the development of algorithms that are suitable for thyroid specimens. The majority of studies referenced above are able to perform adequately when the possible interpretations are limited to binary outcomes, but the interpretation of thyroid FNAB is more complex than the current technologies are able to address. Another major technological problem is the time required to scan cytology specimens. Optimal digital images from cytology specimens require scanning of the cytology preparation in multiple layers, so-called "z-stacking," to recreate the three dimensionality usually seen in cytology specimens. Current commercial scanners available on the market require a long time to scan a slide with multiple z-stacking layers, making it very difficult to implement their use in clinical practice. Additionally, these digital scanners are expensive and there is no real perceivable return of investment at this moment, especially in the absence of validated algorithms. Nonetheless, the commercial success of AI applications in automated cervical screening might provide a roadmap towards development of a similar thyroid FNAB solution.

Conclusion

In this article, we have summarized the significant advancements that have been made in the field of AI applications to thyroid cytopathology. While a significant amount of work has been done, we are only at the dawn of a major paradigm shift in pathology towards digital and computational pathology. As more cytopathologists embrace this new technology, we will begin to define how future pathologists can leverage AI technologies to answer essential clinical questions.

Conflict of Interest Statement

The authors have no conflicts of interest to declare.

Funding Sources

The research reported in this publication was supported in part by the Cancer Center Support Grant of the National Institutes of Health/National Cancer Institute under award number P30CA008748. The content is solely the responsibility of the authors and does not necessarily represent the official views of the National Institutes of Health.

Author Contributions

B.K. and O.L. each contributed to the conceptualization, investigation, procurement of resources, and writing of this article.

References

1 Fuchs TJ, Buhmann JM. Computational pathology: challenges and promises for tissue analysis. Comput Med Imaging Graph. 2011 Oct–Dec;35(7–8):515–30.
2 Louis DN, Feldman M, Carter AB, Dighe AS, Pfeifer JD, Bry L, et al. Computational pathology: a path ahead. Arch Pathol Lab Med. 2016 Jan;140(1):41–50.
3 LeCun Y, Bengio Y, Hinton G. Deep learning. Nature. 2015 May 28;521(7553):436–44.
4 Liu Y, Kohlberger T, Norouzi M, Dahl GE, Smith JL, Mohtashamian A, et al. Artificial intelligence-based breast cancer nodal metastasis detection: insights into the black box for pathologists. Arch Pathol Lab Med. 2019 Jul; 143(7):859–68.
5 Tan GH, Gharib H. Thyroid incidentalomas: management approaches to nonpalpable nodules discovered incidentally on thyroid imaging. Ann Intern Med. 1997 Feb 1;126(3): 226–31.
6 Guth S, Theune U, Aberle J, Galach A, Bamberger CM. Very high prevalence of thyroid nodules detected by high frequency (13 MHz) ultrasound examination. Eur J Clin Invest. 2009 Aug;39(8):699–706.
7 Hegedus L. Clinical practice. The thyroid nodule. N Engl J Med. 2004 Oct 21;351(17): 1764–71.
8 Haugen BR, Alexander EK, Bible KC, Doherty GM, Mandel SJ, Nikiforov YE, et al. 2015 American Thyroid Association management guidelines for adult patients with thyroid nodules and differentiated thyroid cancer: The American Thyroid Association Guidelines Task Force on Thyroid Nodules and Differentiated Thyroid Cancer. Thyroid. 2016 Jan;26(1):1–133.
9 Ho AS, Sarti EE, Jain KS, Wang H, Nixon IJ, Shaha AR, et al. Malignancy rate in thyroid nodules classified as Bethesda Category III (AUS/FLUS). Thyroid. 2014 May;24(5):832–9.
10 Straccia P, Rossi ED, Bizzarro T, Brunelli C, Cianfrini F, Damiani D, et al. A meta-analytic review of the Bethesda System for Reporting Thyroid Cytopathology: has the rate of malignancy in indeterminate lesions been underestimated? Cancer Cytopathol. 2015 Dec; 123(12):713–22.
11 Cibas ES, Ali SZ. The 2017 Bethesda System for Reporting Thyroid Cytopathology. Thyroid. 2017 Nov;27(11):1341–6.
12 Ko YS, Hwang TS, Kim JY, Choi YL, Lee SE, Han HS, et al. Diagnostic limitation of fine-needle aspiration (FNA) on indeterminate thyroid nodules can be partially overcome by preoperative molecular analysis: assessment of RET/PTC1 rearrangement in BRAF and RAS wild-type routine air-dried FNA specimens. Int J Mol Sci. 2017 Apr 12;18(4):806.
13 Zhang M, Lin O. Molecular testing of thyroid nodules: a review of current available tests for fine-needle aspiration specimens. Arch Pathol Lab Med. 2016 Dec;140(12):1338–44.
14 Nishino M, Nikiforova M. Update on molecular testing for cytologically indeterminate thyroid nodules. Arch Pathol Lab Med. 2018 Apr;142(4):446–57.
15 Li F-F, Johnson J, Yeung S. CS231n: convolutional neural networks for visual recognition; 2017.
16 Karakitsos P, Cochand-Priollet B, Pouliakis A, Guillausseau PJ, Ioakim-Liossi A. Learning vector quantizer in the investigation of thyroid lesions. Anal Quant Cytol Histol. 1999 Jun;21(3):201–8.
17 Cochand-Priollet B, Koutroumbas K, Megalopoulou TM, Pouliakis A, Sivolapenko G, Karakitsos P. Discriminating benign from malignant thyroid lesions using artificial intelligence and statistical selection of morphometric features. Oncol Rep. 2006;15(Spec no. 4):1023–6..:
18 Gopinath B, Shanthi N. Support vector machine based diagnostic system for thyroid cancer using statistical texture features. Asian Pac J Cancer Prev. 2013;14(1):97–102.
19 Gopinath B, Shanthi N. Computer-aided diagnosis system for classifying benign and malignant thyroid nodules in multi-stained FNAB cytological images. Australas Phys Eng Sci Med. 2013 Jun;36(2):219–30.
20 Gopinath B, Shanthi N. Development of an automated medical diagnosis system for classifying thyroid tumor cells using multiple classifier fusion. Technol Cancer Res Treat. 2015 Oct;14(5):653–62.
21 Sanyal P, Mukherjee T, Barui S, Das A, Gangopadhyay P. Artificial intelligence in cytopathology: a neural network to identify papillary carcinoma on thyroid fine-needle aspiration cytology smears. J Pathol Inform. 2018;9:43.
22 Guan Q, Wang Y, Ping B, Li D, Du J, Qin Y, et al. Deep convolutional neural network VGG-16 model for differential diagnosing of papillary thyroid carcinomas in cytological images: a pilot study. J Cancer. 2019;10(20): 4876–82.
23 Simonyan K, Zisserman A. Very deep convolutional networks of large-scale image recognition.

24 Szegedy C, Vanhoucke V, Ioffe S, Shlens J, Wojna Z. Rethinking the inception architecture for computer vision. IEEE conference on computer vision and pattern recognition (CVPR). 2016 Jun 27–30. Las Vegas, NV: IEEE; 2016. p. 2818–26.
25 Elliott Range DD, Dov D, Kovalsky SZ, Henao R, Carin L, Cohen J. Application of a machine learning algorithm to predict malignancy in thyroid cytopathology. Cancer Cytopathol. 2020 Apr;128(4):287–95.
26 Zoulias EA, Asvestas PA, Matsopoulos GK, Tseleni-Balafouta S. A decision support system for assisting fine needle aspiration diagnosis of thyroid malignancy. Anal Quant Cytol Histol. 2011 Aug;33(4):215–22.
27 Ippolito AM, De Laurentiis M, La Rosa GL, Eleuteri A, Tagliaferri R, De Placido S, et al. Neural network analysis for evaluating cancer risk in thyroid nodules with an indeterminate diagnosis at aspiration cytology: identification of a low-risk subgroup. Thyroid. 2004 Dec;14(12):1065–71.
28 Shapiro NA, Poloz TL, Shkurupij VA, Tarkov MS, Poloz VV, Demin AV. Application of artificial neural network for classification of thyroid follicular tumors. Anal Quant Cytol Histol. 2007 Apr;29(2):87–94.
29 Savala R, Dey P, Gupta N. Artificial neural network model to distinguish follicular adenoma from follicular carcinoma on fine needle aspiration of thyroid. Diagn Cytopathol. 2018 Mar;46(3):244–9.
30 LiVolsi VA, Baloch Z. Noninvasive follicular tumor with papillary-like nuclear features: a practice changer in thyroid pathology. Arch Pathol Lab Med. 2020 Mar 30.
31 Maleki S, Zandvakili A, Gera S, Khutti SD, Gersten A, Khader SN. Differentiating noninvasive follicular thyroid neoplasm with papillary-like nuclear features from classic papillary thyroid carcinoma: analysis of cytomorphologic descriptions using a novel machine-learning approach. J Pathol Inform. 2019;10:29.

Acta Cytologica

Review

Acta Cytologica 2021;65:330–334
DOI: 10.1159/000513286

Received: August 13, 2020
Accepted: November 4, 2020
Published online: February 23, 2021

Applications of Computational Pathology in Head and Neck Cytopathology

Trang K. Lollie Jeffrey F. Krane

Department of Pathology and Laboratory Medicine, David Geffen School of Medicine at UCLA, Los Angeles, CA, USA

Keywords

Thyroid · Head and neck · Salivary gland · Squamous cell carcinoma · Fine-needle aspiration · Computational analysis

Abstract

Background: The application of computational technology to head and neck cytology material has been explored experimentally in several areas with a variety of potential applications. ***Summary:*** This review summarizes the application of these techniques to the diagnosis of thyroid, salivary gland, and other head and neck fine-needle aspiration specimens. Current limitations and potential future applications in diagnosis are discussed along with the possibilities for therapeutic applications of computational methodology. ***Key Message:*** Particularly promising applications include resolving diagnostic uncertainty in indeterminate thyroid aspirates and assessing the tumor microenvironment in response to immunotherapy for squamous cell carcinoma.

Introduction

Technological advancements in artificial intelligence and machine learning have enabled groundbreaking computational models to support clinical diagnosis and therapeutic decision-making. Integration of machine learning processes such as artificial neural networks (ANNs), deep learning, genetic algorithms, discriminant analysis, and classification and regression trees has been successfully implemented in various sectors of medicine [1]. While light microscopic evaluation remains the gold standard for most pathological diagnosis, the precise measurements and quantification provided by computational analysis promise a degree of objectivity that may help to resolve diagnostic uncertainty in ambiguous cases that are prone to subjective interpretation. Computational methodology also offers the ability to perform and analyze complex iterative tasks in an objective quantifiable manner not possible with routine examination.

The ease with which many head and neck lesions can be accessed via palpation or ultrasound guidance coupled with the capability of rapidly and accurately diagnosing such lesions via minimally invasive fine-needle aspiration (FNA) biopsy have increased cytopathology's footprint in head and neck pathology. Diagnoses are rendered by evaluating individual cells instead of larger tissue biopsies which improves patient safety through reduced procedural complications while also decreasing overall costs. The ability to analyze specific diagnostic cytologic cellular criteria makes cytopathology ideal for computational applications by objectively quantifying morphologic findings. This review will address the efforts and advances

karger@karger.com
www.karger.com/acy

Karger

Jeffrey F. Krane
Department of Pathology and Laboratory Medicine
David Geffen School of Medicine at UCLA
10833 Le Conte Ave., CHS 13-145F, Los Angeles, CA 90095 (USA)
jkrane@mednet.ucla.edu

that have been made in applying digital and computational techniques to head and neck cytology, specifically with regard to thyroid FNA, salivary gland FNA, and head and neck squamous cell carcinoma. Efforts to apply computational cytology for clinical diagnosis and management are summarized, shortcomings of current models are highlighted, and potential future applications are discussed.

Thyroid Lesions

Thyroid FNA is the gold standard diagnostic test for thyroid nodule evaluation. Most thyroid nodules prove to be benign via FNA. For follicular neoplasms, thyroid FNA is primarily a screening test with the majority of cytologically concerning nodules ultimately proving to be benign. In contrast, thyroid FNA can serve as a diagnostic test for papillary thyroid carcinoma (PTC), particularly for classic and tall cell variants in which the cytologic features are usually definitive. Follicular variants of PTC and the indolent noninvasive follicular thyroid neoplasm with papillary-like nuclear features (NIFTP) are more challenging and often result in an indeterminate diagnosis (Bethesda categories III–V). Indeterminate aspirates encompass benign lesions for which surgery could be avoided and neoplasms where lobectomy or near total thyroidectomy would be more appropriate. Accordingly, there is intense interest in resolving diagnostic uncertainty for thyroid nodules with indeterminate cytologic features. Molecular testing has largely filled this role, but an alternative, potentially cost-effective approach is to use computational assistance in an attempt to resolve diagnostic uncertainty.

Computational technology has been applied to thyroid FNA material in numerous studies dating back as far as 1980 [2] (reviewed by Chain et al. [3]). Comparison of these studies is challenging as they vary in the substrate being assessed (smear preparation types and static vs. whole slide images), diagnostic material input (benign, PTC, and follicular carcinoma), parameters being assessed, diagnoses attempting to be distinguished, and the underlying technology implemented to make the assessment. An early proof of concept of computational cytology's diagnostic capabilities was provided in 1996 by Karakitsos et al. [4] using backpropagation in ANNs to improve distinction between benign versus malignant thyroid nuclei. Using image analysis to assess 26 parameters of nuclear morphometry in May-Grünwald-Giemsa-stained smears from 51 specimens (including 12 PTCs and 4 follicular/Hürthle cell carcinomas), correct classification was achieved for 90.6% of nuclei as either benign or malignant. At a single patient level, 98% of cases were classified correctly. In a subsequent larger study, the same group verified that a variety of ANN approaches were superior to a linear classifier approach (87–89% overall accuracy vs. 61%) on an individual case basis. In those cases with an indeterminate cytologic diagnosis, overall accuracy of the ANN was diminished (74–81%) [5].

ANNs have been developed to recognize specific pathological thyroid entities. In 2007, Shapiro et al. [6] applied ANNs to analyze nuclear morphometric parameters (area, perimeter, and shape) and chromatin texture (mean value and standard deviation of gray levels) to differentiate follicular tumors and reported an ability to distinguish follicular adenomas from follicular carcinomas in 87% (73/84) of cases. Convoluted neural networks, a form of ANN that propagates feedforward neural networks of whole image inputs and accordingly categorizes images into specific categories, were tested by Sanyal et al. [7] to separate PTC from non-PTC. Whole images at both ×10 and ×40 magnification were passed through multiple feedforward layers and eventually converted to a binary choice of PTC or non-PTC with a reported sensitivity of 90%, specificity of 83%, and overall accuracy of 85%. However, limitations attributed to potential "overfitting" of training data resulted in findings such as vague papillary formations by normal follicular cells or thick colloid occasionally being misclassified as PTC.

A number of studies have attempted to transform subjective cytologic criteria used in thyroid FNA diagnosis into quantitatively classifiable parameters. Most such studies focus on nuclear parameters that distinguish papillary or follicular carcinomas from benign thyroid nodules. For example, Murata et al. [8] used image analysis and morphological abstraction by factor analysis with combined morphometry and textural parameters to show that PTCs had larger, more irregular nuclei with higher contrast chromatin distribution while follicular carcinomas had larger nuclei with a more monotonous chromatin distribution when compared to their benign counterparts. Overall, nuclear area measurements appear to most reliably distinguish PTC from benign nodules, although other factors related to nuclear shape and chromatin characteristics are predictive in some studies [3, 9–14]. For follicular carcinomas, nuclear size variation may be a more important distinguishing feature [15, 16].

While distinction of clearly benign versus malignant lesions holds academic interest, the ultimate value of quantitative techniques for diagnosis likely rests in how useful they might be in resolving diagnostic uncertainty in challenging cases. Relatively few studies have focused on this issue, particularly since the advent of the use of Bethesda system terminology [3, 17–19]. In one such study, computerized nuclear morphometry was assessed in 9 cytohistologically discordant cases. Two cases originally diagnosed as AUS/FLUS on cytology that proved to be PTC on histopathology exhibited nuclear parameters (such as mean nuclear measurements of diameter, perimeter, and area) closer to those observed in other neoplastic cases. Conversely, 7 false-positive cases originally diagnosed as Bethesda category V or VI that proved to be goiter or lymphocytic thyroiditis histologically exhibited nuclear features comparable to other nonneoplastic cases [17]. In a similar demonstration of the potential value of nuclear morphometry in equivocal cases, Chain et al. [3] analyzed nuclear area and elongation of follicular cells in thyroid FNAs in whole slide images. PTC showed the largest mean and median nuclear area and elongation, whereas benign lesions had the smallest and roundest morphology. Statistically significant differences were identified among indeterminant cases that proved to be benign versus those proving to be PTC. Cases that proved to be NIFTP also differed from PTC cases but exhibited more overlap with benign cases.

In the largest study to date, a machine learning algorithm was used to predict malignancy on whole slide images from 908 cases [19]. The authors used 2 convoluted neural networks, one developed to identify follicular cells and the second to classify aspirates as benign or malignant and to recapitulate Bethesda system classification. The algorithm achieved comparable overall performance to an expert cytopathologist in distinguishing benign and malignant nodules with a sensitivity of 92.0% and a specificity of 90.5%. Since the cytopathologist performed better at the extremes (benign or malignant diagnoses), a combined approach in which the machine learning algorithm was only applied in cytologically indeterminate cases was evaluated and yielded the greatest overall performance. The authors propose that their algorithm could be used in risk stratifying indeterminate aspirates with potential improvements made via modeling that would integrate clinical and ultrasonographic data.

Rather than directly assessing morphologic features, a recent study used a machine learning algorithm to distinguish classic PTC from NIFTP/encapsulated follicular variants of PTC based on microscopic descriptions contained within FNA reports [20]. This method achieved a 76% success rate overall. The authors propose that their approach could be valuable in developing a data-driven scoring system for making this distinction in clinical practice.

To date, most morphometric-based studies in thyroid FNA have been limited by small sample sizes, the need for manual identification and extraction of nuclei for analysis, and long computational times. The more recent use of whole slide imaging promises to facilitate and potentially automate future applications, but a current limitation is the massive storage requirements required which has limited studies thus far to the use of a single slide from each case [3, 19]. Nevertheless, these recent studies suggest that there is significant potential in the near future for using computational technology with machine learning algorithms in refining diagnostic uncertainty in indeterminate cases.

Salivary Gland Lesions

Cytologic diagnosis of salivary gland tumors is especially challenging due to the wide variety of benign and malignant neoplasms described, many of which exhibit extensive morphologic overlap. This complexity in classification suggests that broad cytomorphometric analysis of salivary gland tumors may lack the nuance needed for specific differential diagnostic considerations. Nevertheless, one such attempt exists in the literature in which Obad-Kovacevic et al. [21] applied 13 morphometric parameters to a study of 64 parotid gland tumors. Area, perimeter, convex area, convexity, maximal and minimum radius, length, breadth, form factor, elongation factor, area symmetry factor, and perimeter symmetry factor significantly differed between benign and malignant tumors. Receiver operative characteristic curves of area, perimeter, convex area, maximum radius, length, and form factor were useful in distinguishing benign from malignant tumors. Minimal and maximum radius, convexity, breadth, form factor, and elongation significantly differed in whole cell morphometry parameters. The authors concluded that digital cytomorphometry can assist as an objective tool in distinguishing malignant from benign salivary gland tumors, especially in cases with hypocellular material. Further study is clearly needed, particularly in the context of specific diagnostically challenging scenarios (e.g., basaloid aspirates) to establish whether there is utility for this technology in clinical practice.

Squamous Cell Carcinoma

Some of the most exciting potential applications of computational cytology are in the diagnosis and management of head and neck squamous cell carcinomas. Cytologic diagnosis of squamous cell carcinoma is typically straightforward; however, cystic lesions are often a notable exception where there can be difficulty in distinguishing cystic metastasis of squamous cell carcinoma from a benign developmental cyst due to sample hypocellularity, extensive inflammation, reactive changes, and cellular debris [22]. Image cytometry DNA analysis has been used to assess aneuploidy (defined as DNA values exceeding 5c) to make this distinction both retrospectively [23] and prospectively[24]. In the prospective study, 50 patients with cystic lesions in the neck had aneuploidy identified by DNA analysis in 8/9 cases of cytologically confirmed squamous cell carcinoma metastasis and in all 4 cytologically inconclusive but histologically confirmed cystic metastatic lesions. Esophageal carcinoma accounted for the one discordant diploid case. Conversely, all benign lesions were diploid.

Furthermore, point-of-care technology is being developed to provide immediate feedback of malignant oral lesions that require urgent referral for treatment. In a cytology-on-a-chip approach, brush cytology samples were applied to microfluidic-based cell capture systems, and numeric indices were assigned based on cell phenotypes to determine probability of malignancy [25]. Additional features such as clinical history were also integrated into the program's interface and could be coupled with molecular marker results. These innovative studies demonstrate computational cytology's potential in quickly triaging cases and improving referral efficiency, particularly in settings where cytopathology expertise may not be immediately available.

A recent, potentially groundbreaking application of computational cytology is in the field of cancer immunotherapy surveillance. PD-1/PD-L1 inhibitor immunotherapy has revolutionized the treatment landscape across a multitude of tumor types. Response to PD-1/PD-L1 inhibitors is predicted by monitoring PD-L1 level expressed by tumor cells. However, tumor cells often adapt under treatment pressures and fluidly reshape the tumor microenvironment (TME). The complexity of defining changes in the TME that correlate with treatment responsiveness exceeds the capabilities of routine pathologic evaluation due to the need to evaluate a complex array of parameters and cell types both spatially and temporally. Mapping the TME using computational techniques at the cellular and molecular levels may help identify the next generation of predictive biomarkers and further guide clinical management as the TME evolves over the course of treatment. Cytologic assessment of FNAs is ideal for posttreatment surveillance as it is minimally invasive, cost effective, and allows for frequent serial sampling compared to tissue biopsy. A novel, technologically innovative rapid chemistry-enabled FNA ("FAST-FNA") is currently being evaluated to enable rapid multiplex biomarker analysis using DNA barcode-modified antibodies, ultrafast destaining and "click chemistry" reactions, and automated image cytometry readers [26]. Analogous to the combined positive score used in tissue biopsies, 2 newly developed scores (FAST PD-L1 and FAST cold/hot score) could potentially offer a quicker (approximately 2 h from cell harvesting), more cost effective, and more nuanced alternative to standard PD-L1 assessment that is amenable to serial monitoring. Use of a deep learning-enabled fluorescence cytometer, a stand-alone unit weighing 6 pounds, is currently under clinical investigation.

Conclusion

Despite great promise, significant hurdles remain to the widespread adoption of computational cytology in head and neck cytology specimens. Nuclear morphometric studies typically require tedious and time-consuming manual selection of target nuclei (typically at least 100 nuclei per case). Initial startup requires extensive testing, potentially expensive specialized equipment, and fine-tuning of multiple parametric measurements to determine suitable algorithms. The training process mandates substantial computational power and a large training set to provide enough data for machine learning, which may be prone to data overfitting.

To date, the use of computational cytology in head and neck cytology has largely been limited to the research setting. Extensive literature exists within the area of thyroid cytology, but the technology has yet to establish its ability to provide significant added value in routine practice. Nevertheless, advances in computing power, storage, imaging, and machine learning algorithms point to real potential in the near future for this technology to play a role in resolving diagnostic uncertainty in indeterminate thyroid FNA specimens as an adjunct to routine microscopy and as a potential alternative to molecular testing. Conversely, the complexity of salivary gland tumor diagnosis suggests that computational techniques are unlikely to have a widespread role in the diagnostic realm for these specimens in the foreseeable future. With regard to head and neck squamous cell carcinomas, computational cytology may have potential as a tool in point-of-care testing. The potential application of complex quantitative analysis to evaluate the TME in head and neck squamous cell carcinomas via rapid multiplex biomarker analysis for immunotherapy surveillance holds great theoretical promise. Should this promise be fulfilled, one can readily envision the application of a similar approach to other advanced head and neck malignancies, such as thyroid and salivary gland carcinomas, as well as tumors from other primary sites.

Statement of Ethics

The authors have no ethical conflicts to disclose.

Conflict of Interest Statement

The authors have no conflicts of interest to declare.

Funding Sources

No funding was received.

Author Contributions

T.K.L. and J.F.K.: conception, analysis, drafting, revising, and final approval of work.

References

1 Pouliakis A, Karakitsou E, Margari N, Bountris P, Haritou M, Panayiotides J, et al. Artificial neural networks as decision support tools in cytopathology: past, present, and future. Biomed Eng Comput Biol. 2016 Feb 18;7:1–18.
2 Boon ME, Löwhagen T, Willems JS. Planimetric studies on fine needle aspirates from follicular adenoma and follicular carcinoma of the thyroid. Acta Cytol. 1980;24(2):145–8.
3 Chain K, Legesse T, Heath JE, Staats PN. Digital image-assisted quantitative nuclear analysis improves diagnostic accuracy of thyroid fine-needle aspiration cytology. Cancer Cytopathol. 2019;127(8):501–13.
4 Karakitsos P, Cochand-Priollet B, Guillausseau PJ, Pouliakis A. Potential of the back propagation neural network in the morphologic examination of thyroid lesions. Anal Quant Cytol Histol. 1996;18(6):494–500.
5 Cochand-Priollet B, Koutroumbas K, Megalopoulou TM, Pouliakis A, Sivolapenko G, Karakitsos P. Discriminating benign from malignant thyroid lesions using artificial intelligence and statistical selection of morphometric features. Oncol Rep. 2006;15(4):1023–6.
6 Shapiro NA, Poloz TL, Shkurupij VA, Tarkov MS, Poloz VV, Demin AV. Application of artificial neural network for classification of thyroid follicular tumors. Anal Quant Cytol Histol. 2007;29(2):87–94.
7 Sanyal P, Mukherjee T, Barui S, Das A, Gangopadhyay P. Artificial intelligence in cytopathology: a neural network to identify papillary carcinoma on thyroid fine-needle aspiration cytology smears. J Pathol Inform. 2018;9(1):43.
8 Murata S, Mochizuki K, Nakazawa T, Kondo T, Nakamura N, Yamashita H, et al. Morphological abstraction of thyroid tumor cell nuclei using morphometry with factor analysis. Microsc Res Tech. 2003;61(5):457–62.
9 Sassi I, Mangili F, Sironi M, Freschi M, Cantaboni A. Morphometric evaluation of fine needle biopsy of single thyroid nodules. Pathol Res Pract. 1989;185(5):722–5.
10 Słowińska-Klencka D, Klencki M, Sporny S, Lewiński A. Karyometric analysis in the cytologic diagnosis of thyroid lesions. Anal Quant Cytol Histol. 1997;19(6):507–13.
11 Kirillov VA, Yuschenko YP, Paplevka AA, Demidchik EP. Thyroid carcinoma diagnosis based on a set of karyometric parameters of follicular cells. Cancer. 2001;92(7):1818–27.
12 Harms H, Hofmann M, Ruschenburg I. Fine needle aspiration of the thyroid: Can an image processing system improve differentiation? Anal Quant Cytol Histol. 2002;24(3):147–53.
13 Khatri P, Choudhury M, Jain M, Thomas S. Role of morphometry in the cytological differentiation of benign and malignant thyroid lesions. J Cytol. 2017;34(1):1–4.
14 Deka L, Gupta S, Gupta R, Gupta K, Kaur CJ, Singh S. Nuclear morphometry and texture analysis on cytological smears of thyroid neoplasms: a study of 50 cases. Malays J Pathol. 2017;39(1):33–7.
15 Nagashima T, Suzuki M, Oshida M, Hashimoto H, Yagata H, Shishikura T, et al. Morphometry in the cytologic evaluation of thyroid follicular lesions. Cancer. 1998;84(2):115–8.
16 Savala R, Dey P, Gupta N. Artificial neural network model to distinguish follicular adenoma from follicular carcinoma on fine needle aspiration of thyroid. Diagn Cytopathol. 2018;46(3):244–9.
17 Yashaswini R, Suresh TN, Sagayaraj A. Cytological evaluation of thyroid lesions by nuclear morphology and nuclear morphometry. J Cytol. 2017;34(4):197–202.
18 Celik ZE, Altinay S, Kilinc F, Arslan N, Yilmaz BS, Karabagli P, et al. Using computerized cytomorphometry to distinguish between benign and malignant cases in thyroid fine-needle aspiration cytology. Diagn Cytopathol. 2016;44(11):902–11.
19 Elliott Range DD, Dov D, Kovalsky SZ, Henao R, Carin L, Cohen J. Application of a machine learning algorithm to predict malignancy in thyroid cytopathology. Cancer Cytopathol. 2020;128(4):287–95.
20 Maleki S, Zandvakili A, Gera S, Khutti S, Gersten A, Khader S. Differentiating noninvasive follicular thyroid neoplasm with papillary-like nuclear features from classic papillary thyroid carcinoma: analysis of cytomorphologic descriptions using a novel machine-learning approach. J Pathol Inform. 2019;10(1):29.
21 Obad-Kovačević D, Kardum-Skelin I, Jelić-Puškarić B, Vidjak V, Blašković D. Parotid gland tumors: correlation between routine cytology and cytomorphometry by digital image analysis using conventional and newly introduced cytomorphometric parameters. Diagn Cytopathol. 2013;41(9):776–84.
22 Krane JF. Role of cytology in the diagnosis and management of HPV-associated head and neck carcinoma. Acta Cytol. 2013;57(2):117–26.
23 Nordemar S, Högmo A, Lindholm J, Tani E, Sjöström B, Auer G, et al. The clinical value of image cytometry DNA analysis in distinguishing branchial cleft cysts from cystic metastases of head and neck cancer. Laryngoscope. 2002;112(11):1983–7.
24 Nordemar S, Tani E, Högmo A, Jangard M, Auer G, Munck-Wikland E. Image cytometry DNA-analysis of fine needle aspiration cytology to aid cytomorphology in the distinction of branchial cleft cyst from cystic metastasis of squamous cell carcinoma: a prospective study. Laryngoscope. 2004;114(11):1997–2000.
25 McRae MP, Modak SS, Simmons GW, Trochesset DA, Kerr AR, Thornhill MH, et al. Point-of-care oral cytology tool for the screening and assessment of potentially malignant oral lesions. Cancer Cytopathol. 2020;128(3):207–20.
26 Pai SI, Faquin WC, Sadow PM, Pittet MJ, Weissleder R. New technology on the horizon: fast analytical screening technique FNA (FAST-FNA) enables rapid, multiplex biomarker analysis in head and neck cancers. Cancer Cytopathol. 2020 Aug 25;128(11):782–791.

Research Article

Acta Cytologica

Acta Cytologica 2021;65:335–341
DOI: 10.1159/000510474

Received: May 5, 2020
Accepted: July 13, 2020
Published online: October 6, 2020

Developing a Machine Learning Algorithm for Identifying Abnormal Urothelial Cells: A Feasibility Study

Zhihui Zhang[a] Xinyan Fu[b] Jiwei Liu[c] Zhen Huang[b] Natalia Liu[d] Fengqi Fang[c] Jianyu Rao[d]

[a]Department of Pathology, Cancer Hospital, Chinese Academy of Medical Sciences (CHCAMS), Beijing, China; [b]Division of Medical Technology Development, Hangzhou Zhiwei Information & Technology Ltd., Hangzhou, Hangzhou, China; [c]Department of Oncology, The First Hospital of Dalian Medical University (FHDMU), Dalian, China; [d]Department of Pathology and Laboratory Medicine, David Geffen School of Medicine, UCLA, Los Angeles, CA, USA

Keywords

Machine learning · Digital imaging · Urine cytology · Urothelial carcinoma

Abstract

Introduction: Urine cytology plays an important role in diagnosing urothelial carcinoma (UC). However, urine cytology interpretation is subjective and difficult. Morphogo (ALAB, Boston, MA, USA), equipped with automatic acquisition and scanning, optical focusing, and automatic classification with convolutional neural network has been developed for bone marrow aspirate smear analysis of hematopoietic diseases. The goal of this preliminary study was to determine the feasibility of developing a machine learning algorithm on Morphogo for identifying abnormal urothelial cells in urine cytology slides. ***Methods:*** Thirty-seven achieved abnormal urine cytology slides from cases with the diagnosis of atypical urothelial cells and above (suspicions or positive for UC) were obtained from 1 hospital. A pathologist (J.R.) reviewed the slides and manually selected and annotated representative cells to feed into Morphogo with following categories: benign (urothelial cells, squamous cells, degenerated cells, and inflammatory cells), atypical cells, and suspicious cells. Initial validation of the algorithm was performed on a subset of the original 37 cases. Urine samples from additional 12 unknown cases with various histological diagnoses (6 cases of high-grade urothelial carcinoma (HGUC), 1 case of low-grade urothelial carcinoma (LGUC), 1 case of prostate adenocarcinoma, 1 case of renal cell carcinoma, and 4 cases of non-neoplastic conditions) were collected from another hospital for initial blind testing. ***Results:*** A total of 1,910 benign and 1,978 abnormal (atypical and suspicious) cells from 37 slides were annotated for developing and training of the algorithm. This algorithm was validated on 27 slides that resulted in identification of at least 1 abnormal cell per slide, with a total of 200 abnormal cells, and an average of 7.4 cells per slide. Of the 12 unknown cases tested, the original cytology was positive for tumor cells in 2 HGUC samples. Morphogo was abnormal (atypical or suspicious) for 6 samples from patients with UC, including one with LGUC and one with prostate adenocarcinoma. ***Conclusion:*** Morphogo machine learning algorithm is capable of identifying abnormal urothelial cells. Further validation studies with a larger number of urine samples will be needed to determine if it can be used to assist the cytological diagnosis of UC.

karger@karger.com
www.karger.com/acy

Karger

Jianyu Rao
Department of Pathology and Laboratory Medicine
David Geffen School of Medicine, UCLA 10833 Le Conte Ave.
Los Angeles CA 90095 (USA)
JRao@mednet.ucla.edu

Dr. Fenqi Fang MD PhD
Department Oncology
The First Affiliated Hospital of Dalian Medical University
222 Zhongshan Rd., Dalian 116011 (China)
ffqlj@163.com

Introduction

Urinary bladder cancer is the tenth most common and the 13th deadliest cancer worldwide with an estimated 549,000 new cases (3.0% of global cancer diagnoses) and 200,000 deaths per year (2.1% of global cancer deaths) according to GLOBOCAN 2018 [1]. Bladder cancer is more common in men: the global incidence and mortality rates in men are 9.6 and 3.2 per 100,000, respectively. In comparison, the global incidence and mortality rates in women are 2.4 and 0.9 per 100,000 [1]. In China, the estimated numbers of new cases and deaths for men were 62,100 and 32,900; the estimated numbers of new cases and deaths for women in China that same year were 18,400 and 7,800 [2].

Urothelial carcinoma (UC), previously known as transitional cell carcinoma is the most predominant type of bladder cancer. Over 70% of UC can be detected in early non-muscle invasive stages (Ta or T1). These noninvasive or superficially invasive UCs can be treated by local transurethral resection and/or intravesical agents such as Bacillus Calmette-Guerin with excellent rates of survival [3]. However, the recurrence rate is as high as 30–80% within 5 years of tumor resection. Therefore, early diagnosis and monitoring of recurrence are particularly important for UC. Currently, cystoscopy combined with urine cytology is the main diagnostic method for UC. Although cystoscopy with biopsy is the gold standard, the process is invasive, and it may miss flat high-grade or high-up (upper urinary tract) lesions. Cytology is simple and noninvasive but suffers from low sensitivity, especially for low-grade tumors [4, 5]. While numerous biomarkers have been developed, some of which are commercially available (e.g., fluorescence in situ hybridization, or FISH), the widespread use of these markers in the daily clinic setting is limited due to a variety of reasons, including low specificity and high cost, among others [6].

The main challenges for urine cytological analysis of UC are the subjective nature of the interpretation and lack of uniformity of the diagnosis and reporting. To overcome some of these shortcomings, a Paris System (The Paris System for Reporting Urinary Cytology) was developed and widely used for urine cytological diagnosis of UC [7]. This system provides a useful, quantitative matrix to classify urine cytology into negative, atypical, suspicious, or malignant (mainly high-grade UC) cytological categories based on mainly individual cell morphology. Current preparation of urine cytological slides typically utilizes a liquid-based technique, which usually result in slides with uniform monolayer of cells. This liquid-based preparation, coupled with the adaptation of the Paris system for interpretation and reporting, provides an attractive opportunity to develop and test automatic machine learning tools that may improve the accuracy of urine cytological diagnosis of UC. This study attempts to evaluate Morphogo, a fully automatic system digital scanning instrument armed with high power scanning, optimal focusing, and image acquisition combined with convolutional neural network (CNN) based machine learning, for urine cytological diagnosis of UC.

Materials and Methods

Sample and Slides

We first obtained 37 achieved abnormal urine cytology slides with the diagnosis of atypical urothelial cells (AUCs) and above (suspicious or positive for high-grade urothelial cell carcinoma) from Cancer Hospital, Chinese Academy of Medical Sciences, between October 2018 to March 2019. These slides, each from individual cases with histologically confirmed diagnosis of UC, were used for the initial development and training of the system. These slides were prepared using liquid-based cytology (LBC) technology and Papanicolaou staining. Briefly, 50–100 mL of the patient's second urine sample was collected in the morning. The samples were then fixed with an equal amount of 50% ethanol, centrifuged, and processed using the ThinPrep 2000 processor (Hologic Inc., Boston, MA, USA) according to the standard operating procedure for Papanicolaou staining and cover-slipping [8].

For testing, urine samples from additional 12 cases were collected and processed similar to above procedures from the First Hospital of Dalian Medical University without knowledge of the patient's history of UC. These samples were obtained from March 2019 to April 2019. Table 1 presented patient age, sex, original cytology diagnosis, and final histological diagnosis. Morphogo analysis was performed on these samples independently without the knowledge of the above clinical information.

Instrument

The instrument used in this study was Morphogo (ALAB, Boston, MA, USA), a system that was initially developed for the analysis of bone marrow aspirate smears. Morphogo is an instrument equipped with automated slide scanning, optimal focusing, and automated cell classification using a machine learning tool, CNN. It is a deep-learning neural network consisting of convolutional structures that is able to extract features layer by layer from a single cellular image. A CNN reduces limitations and optimizes process of image recognition, making the machine learning-based system more efficient and accurate. When certain types of cell images are used to train the system, CNN can learn morphological characteristics of different types of cells autonomously. Detailed description of the system is provided in a separate article in this issue [9].

In this study, atypical and malignant urothelial cells annotated in acquired 400× images by the pathologist were used to construct a training dataset. The CNN was trained using the dataset to learn morphological features of abnormal urothelial cells. This formed the foundation for machine-based classification of atypical and suspicious for high-grade malignant urothelial cells.

Table 1. Information of unknown cases analyzed by Morphogo

Case	Gender	Age	Clinical symptoms	Original cytology diagnosis	Morphogo	Histological diagnosis
1	Male	80	Hematuria	See tumor cells	Suspicious	HGUC
2	Male	61	Prostatic cancer	–	Abnormal[a]	Prostatic cancer CA
3	Male	61	Bladder tumor	No tumor cells, highly degenerative cells were found	Suspicious[b]	LGUC
4	Male	81	Bladder tumor	No tumor cells. Individual abnormal cells were found	–	HGUC
5	Male	72	Malignant tumors of the renal pelvis	A few heteromorphic cells	Suspicious	HGUC
6	Male	71	Renal calculus	No tumor cells	–	Renal calculus
7	Male	69	Malignant tumors of the renal pelvis	No tumor cells	–	HGUC
8	Female	–	–	Individual abnormal cells	AUCs	Right renal cyst. Bilateral renal calculi
9	Male	69	Benign prostatic hyperplasia	See tumor cells	Suspicious	HGUC
10	Male	76	Bladder mass, recurrence of bladder cancer after CA	No tumor cells	AUCs	HGUC
11	Male	56	Renal masses	–	–	Right renal carcinoma
12	Male	73	Benign prostatic hyperplasia	Individual abnormal cells	–	Prostatic hyperplasia with inflammation

HGUC, high-grade urothelial carcinoma; LGUC, suspicious for high-grade urothelial carcinoma; AUCs, atypical urothelial cells. [a] One case with prostate adenocarcinoma. [b] One case with LGUC.

Methods

Slide Digitization

The instrument digitized the entire stained urine cytology slides by whole-slide imaging under a ×40 objective with z-stacking. Atypical urothelial cells and cells suspicious for UC were located and framed by the cell selection algorithm embedded in the instrument, and individual cell images were displayed in a gallery.

Manual Annotation of Cells

A cytopathologist (J.R. from UCLA) reviewed all 37 training set of achieved urine slides and manually identified and annotated representative categories of cells including: benign (urothelial cells, squamous cells, degenerated cells, and inflammatory cells), atypical cells, and suspicious cells (for high-grade urothelial carcinoma; HGUC). The Paris system criteria were used to determine atypical or suspicious cells [7]. Atypical cell was annotated if the cell had a nuclear-to-cytoplasmic (N:C) ratio greater than 0.5 with 1 additional criteria (hyperchromasia or irregular chromatin or irregular nuclear contour). A suspicious cell was annotated if the cell had an N:C ratio greater than 0.7 and hyperchromasia with either irregular chromatin or irregular nuclear contours. Cells of undetermined type and interfering substances were excluded. It is important to note that, per the Paris system, the diagnosis of "positive for HGUC" should be made based on the number of suspicious cells present.

Training and Validation of the Algorithm

The neural network of the algorithm could automatically extract the characteristics of different cell types in the cell recognition data set, and training was completed after several iterations and cycles. Likewise, each cell acquired by the instrument was also classified into one of the following categories: benign (including urothelial cells, squamous cells, degenerated cells, and inflammatory cells), atypical cells, and suspicious cells (for HGUC). The performance of the algorithm was validated on 27 slides (2 AUCs, 7 suspicious, and 18 positive HGUC) out of 37 urine cytology samples that were available at the time of analysis, as some of the slides were returned to the hospital for patient care reasons.

Preliminary Testing

An additional 12 cases were collected from The First Hospital of Dalian Medical University for cell identification testing (Table 1). The urine cytology slides were prepared similarly using Thinprep technique (Hologic, Inc., Boston, MA, USA) and stained as described above. Whole-slide scanning of the slides was then performed using the Morphogo instrument to identify abnormal cells with the machine learning-based algorithm described above. The captured cellular images were also framed into the gallery and reviewed blindly by a cytopathologist (J.R.). The Morphogo analysis was performed independently, without the knowledge of cytological and histological diagnosis. The pathological results obtained by histopathological examinations were used as the gold standard,

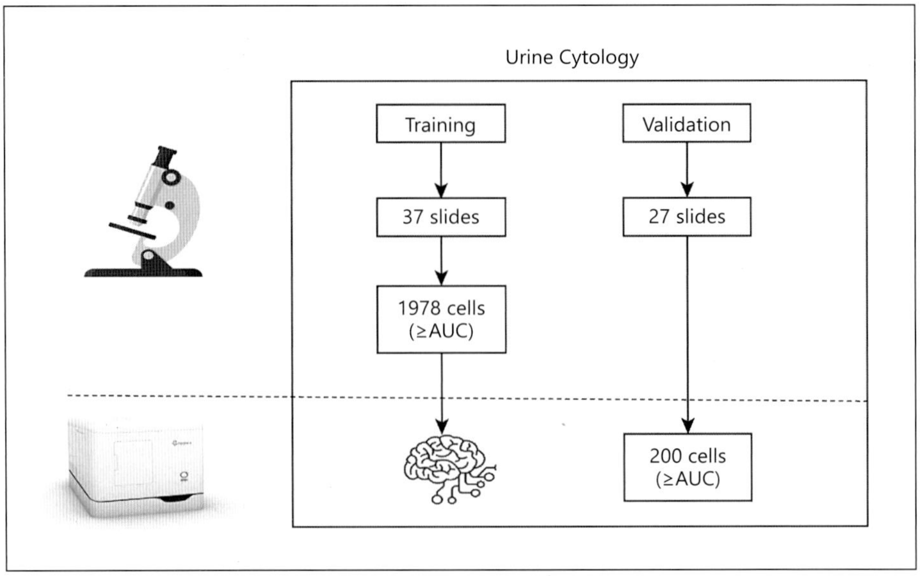

Fig. 1. Diagram of initial training and validation of the Morphogo with urothelial cells. AUCs, atypical urothelial cells.

and the Morphogo findings were compared to the cytology diagnosis.

Statistical Analysis

All analyses were performed using Microsoft Excel 2016 (Microsoft Corporation, Redmond, WA, USA).

Results

Development and Validation of the Algorithm for Cell Classification

A total of 1,978 abnormal (atypical and suspicious for UC) and 1,910 benign cells (urothelial cells, squamous cells, degenerated cells, and inflammatory cells) were manually acquired during the initial training phase of the algorithm (Fig. 1) from a total of 37 abnormal urine cytology slides. These cells were annotated by a single pathologist (J.R.) and fed into the system for training. An algorithm was then established to automatically scan, locate, and identify abnormal urothelial cells. The goal for the algorithm was identification of up to 10 abnormal cells per slide that met the criteria for atypical or suspicious for HGUC. The system will scan all cells in the slide, including inflammatory cells. If 10 abnormal cells were identified, the system would stop the scan and automatically move to the next case. If 10 abnormal cells were not identified, the scan would continue until the entire slide was scanned.

We then validated the algorithm using 27 slides out of the total 37 slides that were still available at the time of analysis. With this strategy, we were able to find at least 1 abnormal cell per slide, with a total of 200 abnormal cells and 226 image fields (400×) acquired by the instrument utilizing the cell classification algorithm, representing an average of 7.4 abnormal cells and 8.4 image fields per slide. These identified cells were loaded into a cell gallery and were reviewed by 1 pathologist (J.R.) in order to confirm that all identified abnormal cells were atypical or suspicious. Figure 2 shows representative images of identified field (Fig. 2a) as well as abnormal urothelial cells (atypical and suspicious Fig. 2b).

Preliminary Test of the Algorithms in Additional Unknown Samples

Of the 12 unknown slides tested, there were 6 slides from 6 individual cases of HGUC, 1 from a case of low-grade UC (LGUC), 1 from a case of prostate adenocarcinoma, 1 from a case of renal cell carcinoma, and 4 from cases with various non-neoplastic conditions (Table 1). The original urine cytology results were positive for tumor cells in 2 HGUC samples, and the urine cytology results analyzed by Morphogo were abnormal (AUCs, suspicious or positive for HGUC) for 6 patients with UC malignancy, including 1 with LGUC (Table 1). The results analyzed by Morphogo were similar to the cytopathologist's diagnosis in case #5 and case #8. However, in case #10, Morphogo found atypical urothelial cells, while the original cytology was negative. Of note, the instrument identified abnormal cells in the cases with prostate adenocarcinoma (case #2) and LGUC (case #3).

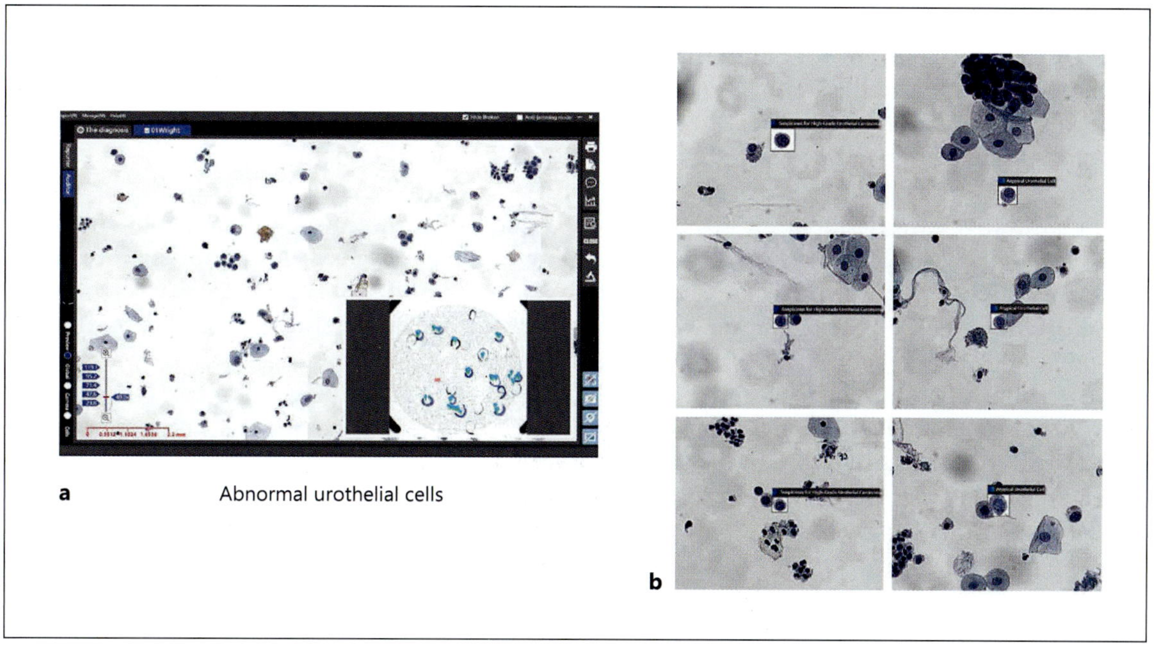

Fig. 2. Representative images of abnormal urothelial cells identified by Morphogo. **a** Identified image field that contained abnormal urothelial cells (×10). **b** Representative examples of identified abnormal urothelial cells (×40). The right panel showed atypical urothelial cells and the left panel showed suspicious urothelial cells. AUCs, atypical urothelial cells.

Discussion/Conclusion

In this study, the instrument Morphogo achieved the goal of automatically scanning urine cytology slides and of performing machine learning-based identification of abnormal urothelial cells (atypical or suspicious for UC) from the scanned images. Preliminary testing of a small number of unknown urine samples showed that such a system is similar to, if not more sensitive than, human cytological evaluation. Interestingly, the instrument also found abnormal cells in the cases of prostate adenocarcinoma and LGUC.

Hematuria is the most common clinical manifestation of bladder cancer patients, and it is the first symptom in approximately 80–90% of patients [2]. At present, urine cytology is the most widely method for evaluating patients with hematuria for the initial diagnosis of UC, as well as monitoring UC patients for the recurrence [5]. The overall sensitivity of urine cytology for the diagnosis of UC ranges from 13 to 75%, and a specificity of 85–100% [2]. Urine cytology has relatively high diagnostic specificity for HGUC [10, 11], but a low sensitivity in general, especially for LGUC [12]. By definition, tumor cells of LGUC have similar individual cell morphological characteristics to normal urothelial cells, which is difficult to distinguish with the human eye. In many countries, urine cytology is not routinely performed as a diagnostic test for UC due to a lack of well-trained and experienced cytopathologist who can perform diagnostic evaluation. Therefore, the diagnosis of UC is almost entirely made by cystoscopy examination, which is not only invasive but also known to miss many high-grade aggressive "flat lesions," including carcinoma in situ, invasive carcinoma, or upper tract lesions. While carcinoma in situ is a precancerous lesion in other organ systems, its presence in the urothelial system is considered a form of a high-grade aggressive and malignant tumor.

LBC effectively improved the sensitivity in clinical diagnosis of UC. LBC was developed in the late 1990s for cell smear and is widely used in cytological assays [13]. Compared to traditional urinary tract cytology, it offers improved slide quality [14] and provides better detection of malignant cells in the urine of patients with bladder tumors [15, 16] while also retaining the high specificity of urine cytology [14, 17]; its pooled sensitivity is 0.58 (0.51–0.65) and its specificity is 0.96 (0.93–0.98) [18].

Slides prepared by LBC, especially ThinPrep (Hologic Inc., Boston, MS, USA), are uniquely prone to individual

Acta Cytologica 2021;65:335–341
DOI: 10.1159/000510474

cell-based digital machine learning analysis, as the slides are typically a monolayer with minimum cellular overlap. Both the LBC slide and the standardized Paris system for reporting urinary cytology provide the backbone for developing digitalized machine learning strategies [7, 19]. The Paris system includes specific diagnostic categories and quantitative criteria for cell morphology to classify cells into atypical urothelial cells, suspicious, and malignant categories. Since a definitive diagnosis of HGUC is based on the number of cells that meet the categories of "suspicious for malignancy" category, this study classified each abnormal individual as either atypical or suspicious. It is interesting to note that Morphogo identified a case of LGUC and a case of prostate adenocarcinoma as suspicious and abnormal, respectively. It is possible though that this case may contain a component of HGUC, and one may need to review of the histology to rule out such a possibility. It is intriguing that Morphogo identified abnormal cells in the urine cytology slides from a patient with prostate adenocarcinoma. Reviewed of this particular slide by cytologist (J.R.) indeed confirmed that these were malignant cells, but whether the cells were urothelial or prostate origin was difficult to determine morphologically.

There are, however, several potential limitations of the current Morphogo system for urine cytology. First, the system was trained entirely to identify individual cell based on the cell classification scheme derived from Paris system. Thus, cells in overlapping clusters or papillary structures may not be analyzed. Further, background features that may affect cellular morphology, such as background inflammation, are not included in the algorithm development. Third, the system was developed and tested on Thinprep slides. Use the system for other type of cytology slides such as Cytospin or Surepath may be challenging as those slides typically contain more overlapping cell. This is a proof-of-concept study with the aim to determine if a machine learning algorithm on the Morphogo system can be developed to identify abnormal urothelial cell, thereby to be used for assisting cytological diagnosis of UC down the road. For this feasibility study, a total of 3,888 individual cells, including 1,910 abnormal and 1,978 normal cells, were identified and annotated to train the system. We demonstrated that the system can effectively detect abnormal cells from the slide based on a small number of urine cytology cases. However, the actual clinical validation will require a much larger number of urine case samples. Another limitation of the study was only 1 pathologist performed annotation of cells during the training phase, which may create bias for subsequent cell classification. For the future clinical validation studies, we expect a team of cytopathologists will be assembled.

Overall, the Morphogo system, which combines fully automatic digital scanning with CNN-based machine learning, can potentially be used to identify abnormal urothelial cells. Although these results may lead to speculation that the machine learning Morphogo system may be able to detect subtle abnormalities beyond the capabilities of the human eye, such a notion can only be tested in larger studies. Multicenter trials are warranted to further demonstrate the efficacy of this system for assisting the cytological diagnosis of UC in a clinical setting, especially in countries where experienced cytopathologists are limited.

Acknowledgements

The authors also would like to thank Xinyi Cao, Kai Huang, Shun Li, Jiajia Hu, Yongtao Liu, and Chenglin Ji from Zhi-Wei Information & Technology, Ltd. for technical assistance.

Statement of Ethics

The project received exemption at the Institutional Review Board for human research subjects at CHCAM and FHDMU each separately, as the study only used achieved urine slides/samples, and no patient identification information was collected and analyzed.

Conflict of Interest Statement

Jianyu Rao received travel support from Zhi-Wei Information & Technology, Ltd. All the other authors declare that they have no conflict of interest.

Funding Sources

This work was supported by ALABS Inc. and Hangzhou Zhi-Wei Information & Technology, Ltd.

Author Contributions

Jianyu Rao and Fengqi Fang conceptualized the study and together with Zhihui Zhang and Jiwei Liu designed the study. Jianyu Rao also led the effort to perform cell classification of urine samples manually. Zhihui Zhang and Fengqi Fang collected urine samples and raw data including patient's histological diagnosis. Xinyan Fu, Zhen Huang, and Natalia Liu provided the technical support and carried out the analysis. The first manuscript was written by Zhihui Zhang, then edited and improved by Jiwei Liu, Natalia Liu, Fengqi Fang, and Jianyu Rao.

References

1 Bray F, Ferlay J, Soerjomataram I, Siegel RL, Torre LA, Jemal A, et al. Global cancer statistics 2018: GLOBOCAN estimates of incidence and mortality worldwide for 36 cancers in 185 countries. CA Cancer J Clin. 2018; 68(6):394–424.

2 China NHCotPsRo. Diagnostic and therapeutic guidelines for bladder cancer. 2018 ed. National Health Committee of the People's Republic of China: Office of the National Health Committee; 2018.

3 Saginala K, Barsouk A, Aluru JS, Rawla P, Padala SA, Barsouk A, et al. Epidemiology of bladder cancer. Medical Sciences. 2020;8(1):15.

4 Manna AK, Sarkar M, Bandyopadhyay U, Chakrabarti S, Pathak S, Sarkar DK, et al. Cytological and morphometric study of urinary epithelial cells with histopathological correlation. Indian J Surg. 2014 Feb;76(1):26–30.

5 Mushtaq J, Thurairaja R, Nair R. Bladder cancer. Surgery. 2019;37(9):529–37.

6 Bhat A, Ritch C. Urinary biomarkers in bladder cancer: where do we stand? Current Opinion in Urology. 2019 Mar 01;29:1.

7 Rosenthal DL, Wojcik EM, Kurtycz DFI. The Paris system for reporting urinary cytology. Springer; 2015.

8 VandenBussche CJ, Rosenthal DL, Olson MT. Adequacy in voided urine cytology specimens: the role of volume and a repeat void upon predictive values for high-grade urothelial carcinoma. Cancer Cytopathol. 2016 Mar; 124(3):174–80.

9 Lu J, Rao A. Morphogo system a tool for computational cytology. Acta Cytologica. 2020.

10 Murphy WM. Current status of urinary cytology in the evaluation of bladder neoplasms. Hum Pathol. 1990 Sep;21(9):886–96.

11 Tone K, Kojima K, Hoshiai K, Kumagai N, Kijima H, Kurose A, et al. An ancillary method in urine cytology: nucleolar/nuclear volume ratio for discrimination between benign and malignant urothelial cells. Diagn Cytopathol. 2016 Jun;44(6):483–91.

12 McCroskey Z, Pambuccian SE, Kleitherms S, Antic T, Cohen MB, Barkan GA, et al. Accuracy and interobserver variability of the cytologic diagnosis of low-grade urothelial carcinoma in instrumented urinary tract cytology specimens. Am J Clin Pathol. 2015 Dec; 144(6):902–8.

13 Nasuti JF, Tam D, Gupta PK. Diagnostic value of liquid-based (Thinprep) preparations in nongynecologic cases. Diagn Cytopathol. 2001 Feb;24(2):137–41.

14 Son SM, Koo JH, Choi SY, Lee HC, Lee YM, Song HG, et al. Evaluation of urine cytology in urothelial carcinoma patients: a comparison of CellprepPlus® liquid-based cytology and conventional smear. Korean J Pathol. 2012 Feb;46(1):68–74.

15 Kapoor K, Datta C, Pal DK. Is liquid-based cytology an alternative to conventional cytology for detection of malignant cells in urine of bladder cancer? Eastern Indian prospective observational study. Turk J Urol. 2019 Sep; 45(5):351–6.

16 Zhang JS, Yuan Q, Hong-Lei AN. Application of thin-prep cytology test in the diagnosis of postoperative recurrence of carcinoma of urinary bladder. Beijing Med J. 2011.

17 Yamashiro K, Taira K, Nakajima M, Azuma M, Koseki M, Abe T, et al. Voided urine cytology and low-grade urothelial neoplasia of the bladder: factors that influence the sensitivity. J Am Soc Cytopathol. 2016 Jul 01;5(4):227–34.

18 Luo Y, She DL, Xiong H, Yang L, Fu SJ. Diagnostic value of liquid-based cytology in urothelial carcinoma diagnosis: a systematic review and meta-analysis. PLoS One. 2015; 10(8):e0134940.

19 Cowan ML, VandenBussche CJ. The paris system for reporting urinary cytology: early review of the literature reveals successes and rare shortcomings. J Am Soc Cytopathol. 2018 Jul 01;7(4):185–94.

Acta Cytologica

Research Article

Acta Cytologica 2021;65:342–347
DOI: 10.1159/000515379

Received: November 10, 2020
Accepted: February 2, 2021
Published online: April 30, 2021

Digital/Computational Technology for Molecular Cytology Testing: A Short Technical Note with Literature Review

Robert Y. Osamura[a, b] Naruaki Matsui[a] Masato Kawashima[a] Hiroyasu Saiga[c] Maki Ogura[c] Tomoharu Kiyuna[c]

[a]Department of Diagnostic Pathology Nippon Koukan Hospital, Kawasaki, Japan; [b]Keio University School of Medicine, Tokyo, Japan; [c]Digital Healthcare Business Development Office, NEC Corp, Tokyo, Japan

Keywords

Digital cytopathology · Artificial intelligence · Molecular cytopathology

Abstract

This short article describes the method of digital cytopathology using Z-stack scanning with or without extended focusing. This technology is suitable to observe such thick clusters as adenocarcinoma on cytologic specimens. Artificial intelligence (AI) has been applied to histological images, but its application on cytologic images is still limited. This article describes our attempt to apply AI technology to cytologic digital images. For molecular analysis, cytologic materials, such as smear, LBC, and cell blocks, have been successfully used for targeted single gene detection and multiplex gene analysis with next-generation sequencing. As a future perspective, the system can be connected to full automation by combining digital cytopathology with AI application to detect target cancer cells and to perform molecular analysis. The literature review is updated according to the subjects.

Introduction

Digital pathology has been used for primary histopathology diagnosis [1, 2]. And these scanned images are used for image analyses, which include histology, immunohistochemistry, and quantitative tissue morphometrics [3–5]. Digitalization of cytology images has been attempted, and now the digital images are successfully used for cytological diagnosis and various analyses [6–9]. Applications of digital cytopathology have been done with Z-stacks because not infrequently neoplastic cells form thick clusters that are difficult to scan with only 1 plane. Summation of these individual planes is called as "extended focusing" [9] and can be applied successfully to observe thickened cell clusters such as adenocarcinomas.

Applications of artificial intelligence (AI) technologies have been attempted mostly in digital histopathology, and its applications in digital cytopathology are very limited [10–14]. For molecular analysis, companion diagnostics, and next-generation sequencing, FFPE materials have been used as standard procedures. Recently, cytologic materials such as smears, LBC, and cell blocks have been successfully used for the above molecular analyses

karger@karger.com
www.karger.com/acy

Karger
OPEN ACCESS

Correspondence to:
Robert Y. Osamura, osamura@keio.jp

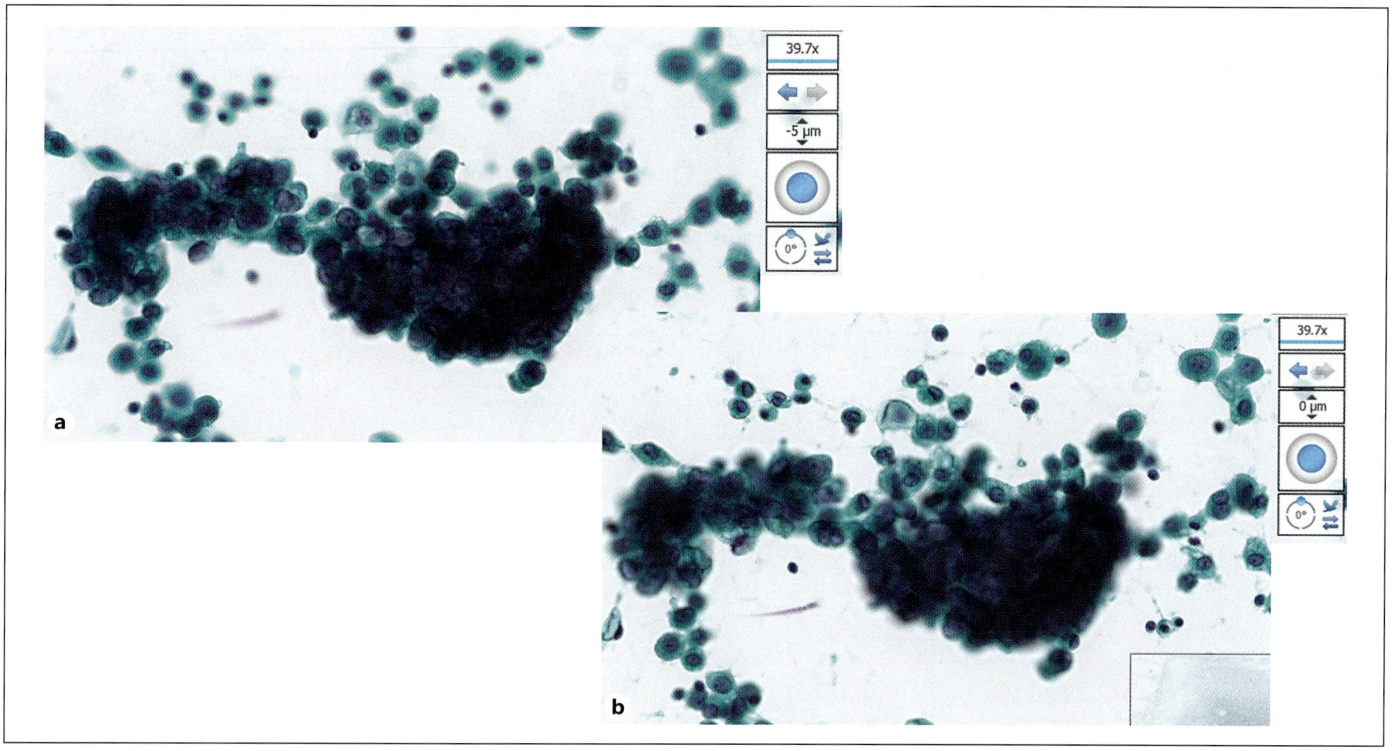

Fig. 1. Z-stack view of adenocarcinoma clusters in the pleural fluid. **a** −5 µm. **b** 0 µm.

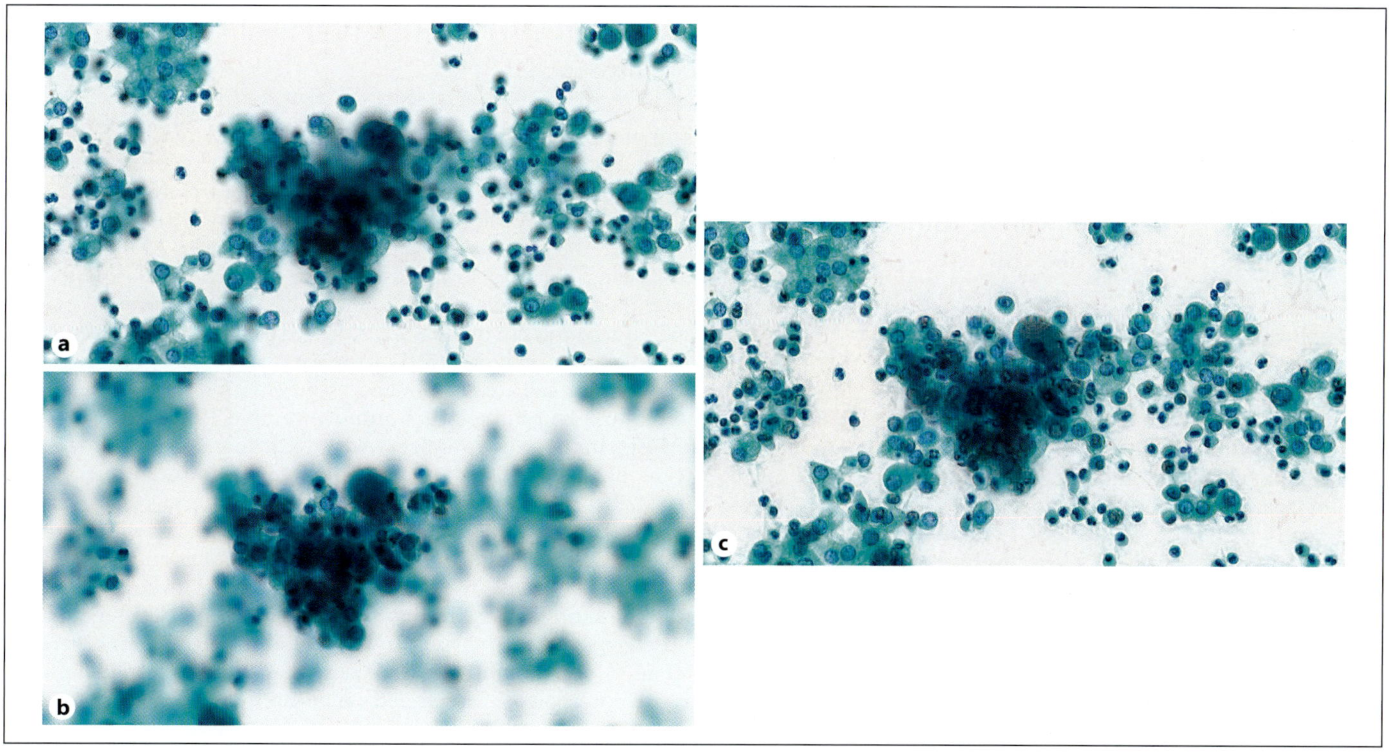

Fig. 2. Z-stack images of adenocarcinoma aggregates in the pleural fluid. The adenocarcinoma cells in particular planes are in focus (**a**, **b**). Extended focusing (**c**) indicates that adenocarcinoma cells in all planes are in focus.

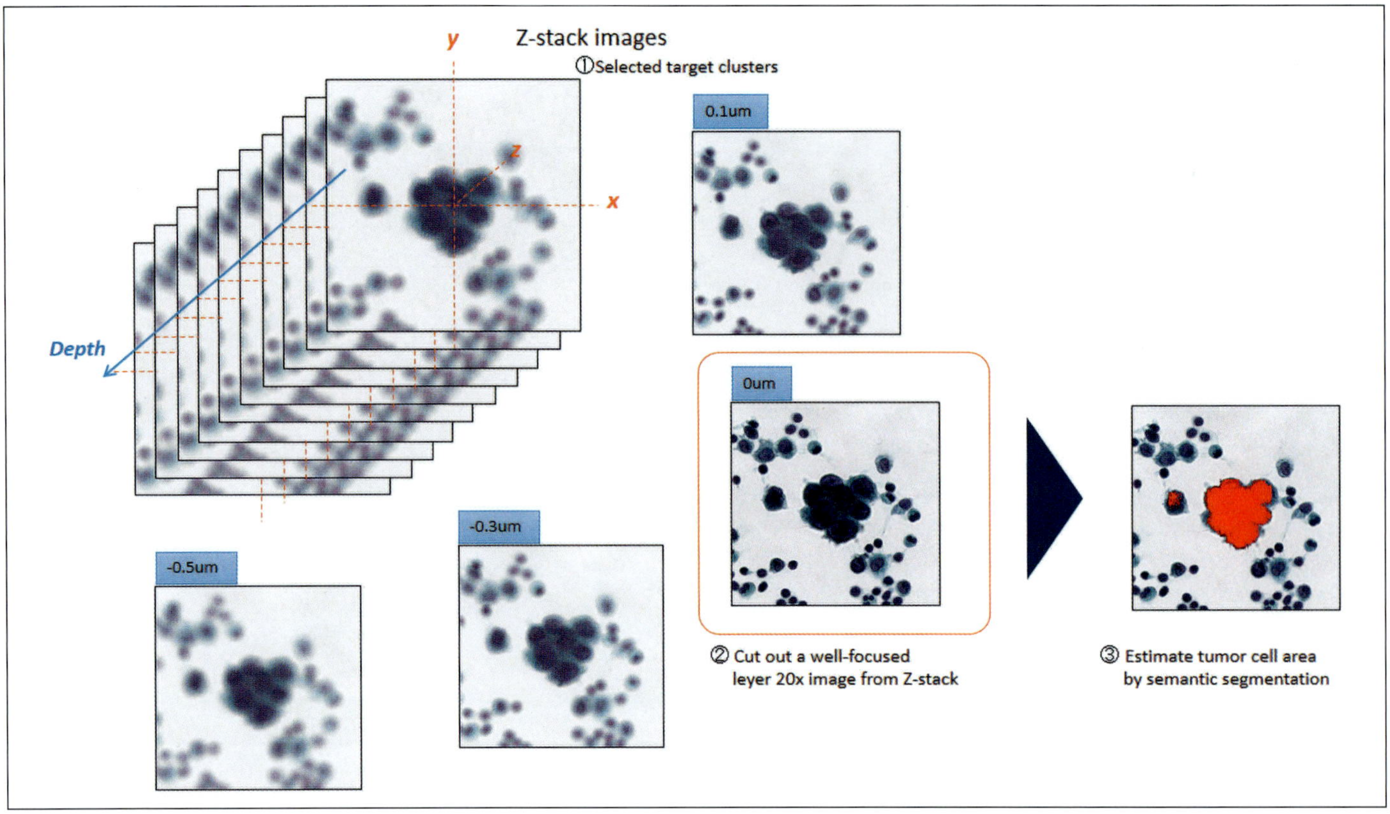

Fig. 3. Application of the AI system to the adenocarcinoma cells in Z-stack ① on 1 plane. The carcinoma cells ② can be detected individually or in clusters ③. Papanicolaou stain. AI, artificial intelligence.

[15–19]. This article was aimed at demonstrating the application of AI technologies to digitized cytopathology images and to the utilization of selected tumor cells for molecular analysis.

Design and Methods

Digital Cytopathology and Application of AI Technologies

Cytologic smears of a total of 6 cases of pleural fluids with metastatic adenocarcinoma of the lung were scanned by NanoZoomer S210 (Hamamatsu Photonics KK, Shizuoka) with Z-stack focusing at 1 µm from −5 µm to +5 µm. The scanning time for samples 1–6 were 5 m 18 s, 16 m 28 s, 13 m 32 s, 14 m 52 s, 19 m 1 s, and 14 m 11 s (m: minutes, s: seconds), respectively.

Thick clusters of lung adenocarcinoma cells are well illustrated by Z-stack scanning. The images captured by NanoZoomer S210 are illustrated in Fig. 1. These individually focused images of different planes can be put together into 1 plane with "all levels are in focus"; this is designated as "extended focusing." This function is saved in the scanner 3DHISTECH (Fig. 2). For the AI applications, Z-stack images of the 6 cases were used as illustrated (Fig. 3).

Image analysis was conducted by means of the technologies developed by NEC Corporation for digital pathology, including annotation schemes, feature extraction, and machine learning such as convolutional neural network [20, 21]. This system successfully detects the areas of gastric adenocarcinomas on tissue sections [20]. We applied these techniques to cytologic materials to detect the cancer cells. The analysis method for AI included the following. (1) Target cell clusters were selected by an experienced pathologist (a single cluster contains 20–30 cells in average). (2) A 20× image was cut out in a well-focused 0-level Z-stack layer of the Whole Slide Imaging. (3) For the extracted image, we estimated each tumor cell area by semantic segmentation (pixel-level classification). To estimate each tumor, we used U-Net with a 256 × 256-px input size (optimizer: Adam, learning rate 10^{-4}, loss function: BCE Dice Loss; data augmentation: flip and color variations) [22, 23].

By applying these AI methods mentioned above, the system detected most of the clusters of adenocarcinoma on the captured images. The images were captured with ×20 magnification (Fig. 3). As an example, these technologies detected small clusters of adenocarcinoma of the lung in the pleural fluid as demonstrated (Fig. 4). Many lymphocytes, macrophages, and mesothelial cells were not labeled. The selected adenocarcinoma cells can be annotated on the images. Exceptionally, a few overlapping and darkly stained cells, probably histiocytes or mesothelial cells, were detected as suspicious for "positive" cells.

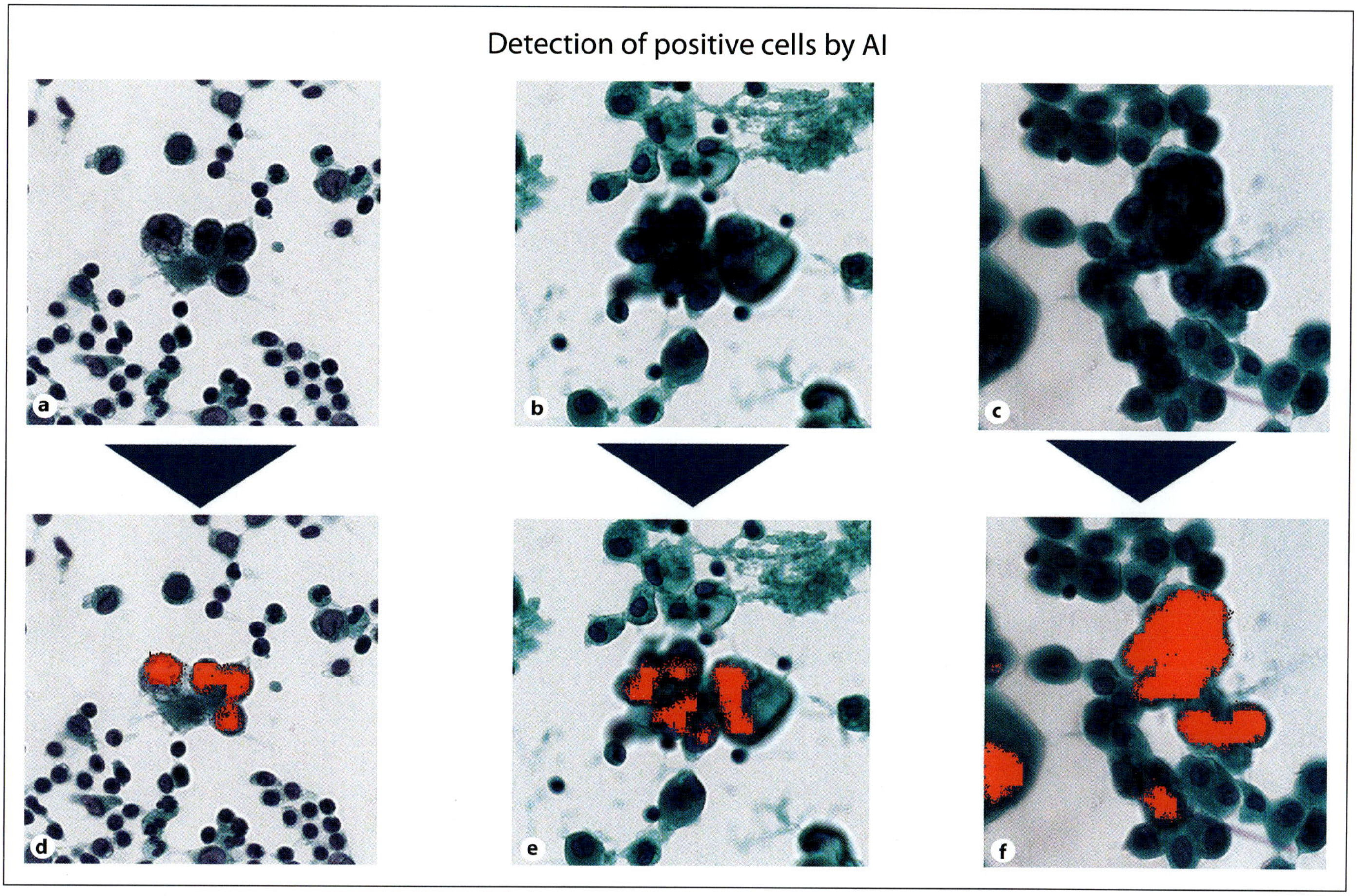

Fig. 4. By applying the AI system to Pap-stained smears of the pleural fluid, various shapes and sizes of clusters of carcinoma cells can be detected (red: adenocarcinoma cells). Lymphocytes (**a**, **d**), histiocytes (**b**, **e**) and mesothelial cells (**c**, **f**) are not labeled. The cancer cells by Papanicolaou stain (**a–c**) are detected by AI application (**d–f**) (in red). AI, artificial intelligence.

A recent literature review on the AI in cytopathology showed the applications of AI on thyroid, urine, pancreaticobiliary, and lung specimens [24]. For the pleural fluid, the detection rate of carcinoma cells by AI was very high, that is, sensitivity and specificity, 100% respectively [23].

Molecular Cytopathology of Cytologic Materials

Using the same cytologic materials as those scanned with Z-stacks, selected clusters of adenocarcinoma cells were subjected to molecular analysis, for example, EGFR mutations, that is, point mutation and deletion. The selected and marked clusters of adenocarcinoma were microdissected (scraped off) manually (Fig. 5) after removing coverslips, and the following molecular analyses were done. In brief, the cells in microtubes were subjected to heat-block at 75° and proteinase *K* treatment for >1 h, and subsequently DNA was extracted by Maxwell® 16 AS2000 (Promega). We used SNP-based mutation detection using i-densy® (Arkray, Japan) [25, 26]. This equipment can detect 3 mutations at a time, such as EGFR exon 21 L858R, exon 19 deletion, and exon 20 T790M, on the same specimen.

The microdissected carcinoma clusters were analyzed by i-densy®, and the mutations in EGFR gene were successfully detected (Fig. 5). By using this method, minimally required numbers of carcinoma cells were calculated as 30 (unpublished data).

Discussion and Conclusion

Computational and Molecular Cytopathology: Current and Future Perspectives

Our results showed promising results for cytopathology by applying a previously established AI system on histologic sections [20]. This system could be applied for the limited target of the cells, which are adenocarcinomas of the lung in the pleural fluid. The system detects the atypical cells, most of which are adenocarcinoma cells, individually or in clusters. But some overlapping non-

Acta Cytologica 2021;65:342–347
DOI: 10.1159/000515379

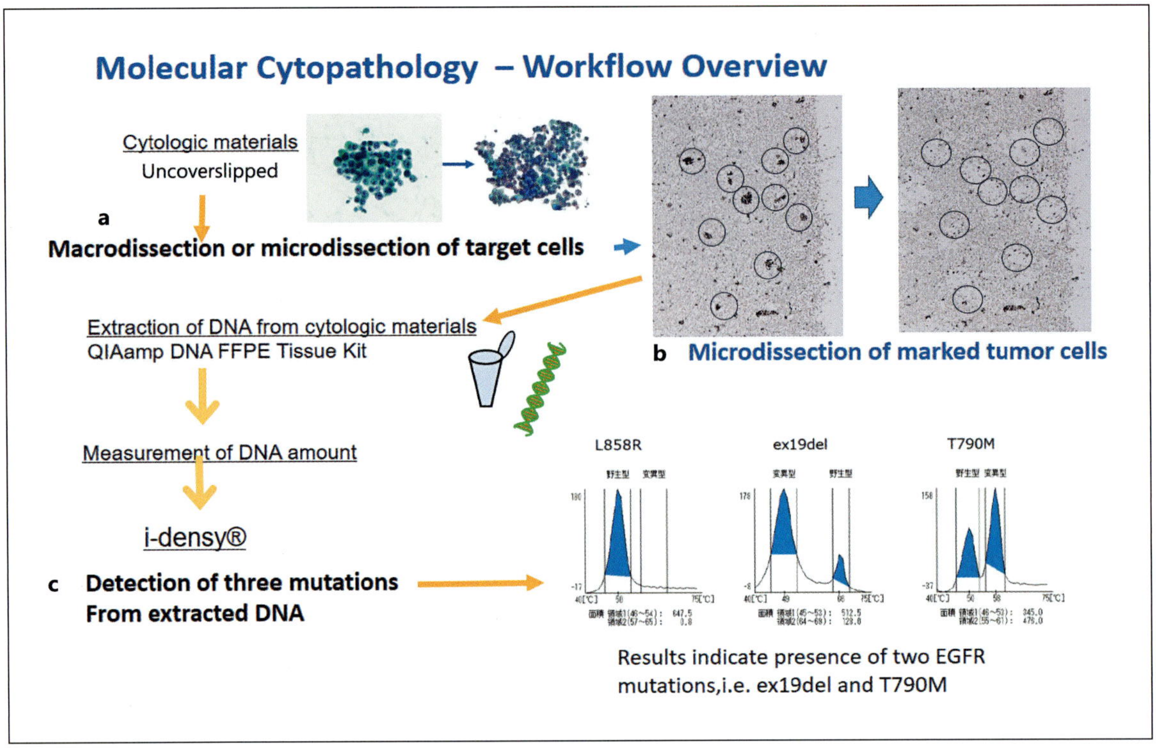

Fig. 5. Workflow from removal of coverslips (**a**), to microdissection (**b**) and submission to i-densy® to analyze EGFR mutation (**c**) after extraction of DNA from cancer cell clusters. Mutational analysis demonstrates 2 different point mutations (EGFR mutation exon 19 del and exon 20 T790M) in the circled adenocarcinoma cells.

neoplastic cells or more darkly stained cells such as histiocytes or mesothelial cells, respectively, were detected as suspicious for malignant cells. This system requires more cases with deep learning and machine learning in order to improve its detection accuracy. For molecular pathology detection, these marked (annotated) cell clusters were microdissected manually and could be used to detect specific genomic changes, mutations, and deletions. Semi-automated laser capture microdissection of cytology samples such as adenocarcinoma of the lung has been reported [27]. It is expected to apply this technology to microdissect the target cancer cells for molecular analysis.

When the AI system and microdissection of the selected target cells could be unified, the fully automated system from the scanning of cytologic specimens to the molecular analysis could be accomplished. It is expected that this fully automated system would be a very efficient system, particularly when the targeted cancer cells are extremely small in number.

Acknowledgements

The authors wish to thank Hamamatsu Photonics, Shizuoka, and e-path Ltd. Co. for their excellent technical support in digitization of cytologic specimens. Part of this study was presented at the 20th International Congress of Cytology (ICC) in Sydney 2019.

Statement of Ethics

This study is the collaboration between Nippon Koukan Hospital and NEC Corp. and has been approved by the Ethical Committees at Nippon Koukan Hospital.

Conflict of Interest Statement

The authors do not have any conflict of interest statement to declare regarding this study.

Funding Sources

The authors have received no funding to pursue this study.

Author Contributions

Robert Y. Osamura: digital cytology and molecular cytology. Naruaki Matsui: micro- and macrodissection of target cancer cells. Masato Kawashima: molecular cytology and technical support. Hiroyasu Saiga: digital cytology and AI application. Maki Ogura: digital cytology and AI application. Tomoharu Kiyuna: digital cytology and AI application.

References

1 Abels E, Pantanowitz L, Aeffner F, Zarella MD, van der Laak J, Bui MM, et al. Computational pathology definitions, best practices, and recommendations for regulatory guidance: a white paper from the digital pathology association. J Pathol. 2019 Nov;249(3):286–94.

2 Zarella MD, Bowman D, Aeffner F, Farahani N, Xthona A, Absar SF, et al. A practical guide to whole slide imaging: a white paper from the digital pathology association. Arch Pathol Lab Med. 2019 Feb;143(2):222–34.

3 Madabhushi A, Lee G. Image analysis and machine learning in digital pathology: challenges and opportunities. Med Image Anal. 2016 Oct;33:170–5.

4 Aeffner F, Zarella MD, Buchbinder N, Bui MM, Goodman MR, Hartman DJ, et al. Introduction to digital image analysis in whole-slide imaging: a white paper from the digital pathology association. J Pathol Inform. 2019; 10:9.

5 Pell R, Oien K, Robinson M, Pitman H, Rajpoot N, Rittscher J, et al. The use of digital pathology and image analysis in clinical trials. J Pathol Clin Res. 2019 Apr;5(2):81–90.

6 Van Es SL, Kumar RK, Pryor WM, Salisbury EL, Velan GM. Cytopathology whole slide images and adaptive tutorials for senior medical students: a randomized crossover trial. Diagn Pathol. 2016 Jan 8;11:1.

7 Wilbur DC. Digital pathology and its role in cytology education. Cytopathology. 2016 Oct; 27(5):325–30.

8 Hanna MG, Pantanowitz L. Reply to why is digital pathology in cytopathology lagging behind surgical pathology? Cancer. 2017 Jul; 125(9):732–20.

9 Capitanio A, Dina RE, Treanor D. Digital cytology: a short review of technical and methodological approaches and applications. Cytopathology. 2018 Aug;29(4):317–25.

10 Tizhoosh HR, Pantanowitz L. Artificial intelligence and digital pathology: challenges and opportunities. J Pathol Inform. 2018;9:38.

11 Bera K, Schalper KA, Rimm DL, Velcheti V, Madabhushi A. Artificial intelligence in digital pathology: new tools for diagnosis and precision oncology. Nat Rev Clin Oncol. 2019 Nov;16(11):703–15.

12 Chang HY, Jung CK, Woo JI, Lee S, Cho J, Kim SW, et al. Artificial intelligence in pathology. J Pathol Transl Med. 2019 Jan;53(1): 1–12.

13 Colling R, Pitman H, Oien K, Rajpoot N, Macklin P; et al. Artificial intelligence in digital pathology: a roadmap to routine use in clinical practice. J Pathol. 2019 Oct;249(2): 143–50.

14 Serag A, Ion-Margineanu A, Qureshi H, McMillan R, Saint Martin MJ, Diamond J, et al. Translational AI and deep learning in diagnostic pathology. Front Med. 2019;6:185.

15 Rossi ED, Schmitt F. Pre-analytic steps for molecular testing on thyroid fine-needle aspirations: the goal of good results. Cytojournal. 2013 Nov 28;10:24.

16 Layfield LJ, Roy-Chowdhuri S, Baloch Z, Ehya H, Geisinger K, Hsiao SJ, et al. Utilization of ancillary studies in the cytologic diagnosis of respiratory lesions: the papanicolaou society of cytopathology consensus recommendations for respiratory cytology. Diagn Cytopathol. 2016 Dec;44(12):1000–9.

17 Jain D, Roy-Chowdhuri S. Molecular pathology of lung cancer cytology specimens: a concise review. Arch Pathol Lab Med. 2018 Sep; 142(9):1127–33.

18 Lozano MD, Echeveste JI, Abengozar M, Mejías LD, Idoate MA, Calvo A, et al. Cytology smears in the era of molecular biomarkers in non-small cell lung cancer: doing more with less. Arch Pathol Lab Med. 2018 Mar;142(3): 291–8.

19 Roy-Chowdhuri S, Dacic S, Ghofrani M, Illei PB, Layfield LJ, Lee C, et al. Collection and handling of thoracic small biopsy and cytology specimens for ancillary studies: guideline from the college of American Pathologists in Collaboration with the American College of chest physicians, Association for Molecular Pathology, American Society of Cytopathology, American Thoracic Society, Pulmonary Pathology Society, Papanicolaou Society of Cytopathology, Society of Interventional Radiology, and Society of thoracic radiology. Arch Pathol Lab Med. 2020 May 13. http://dx.doi.org/10.5858/arpa.2020-0119-CP.

20 Cosatto E, Laquerre PF, Malon C, Graf HP, Saito A, Kiyuna T, et al. Automated gastric cancer diagnosis on H and E-stained sections; training a classifier on large scale with multiple instance machine learning. Medical Imaging 2013: Digital Pathology. 2013;8676: 867605.

21 Malon CD, Cosatto E. Classification of mitotic figures with convolutional neural networks and seeded blob features. J Pathol Inform. 2013;4:9.

22 Nadeem A, Bhuyan M, Shaik A. A review on semantic segmentation from a modern perspective. In: 2019 International Conference on Electrical, Electronics and computer engineering (UPCON). Aligarh, India; 2019. p. 1–6.

23 Ronneberger O, Fischer P, Brox T. U-net: convolutional networks for biomedical image segmentation. International Conference on Medical image computing and computer-assisted intervention. Cham: Springer; 2015. p. 234–41.

24 Landau MS, Pantanowitz L. Artificial intelligence in cytopathology: a review of the literature and overview of commercial landscape. J Am Soc Cytopathol. 2019 Jul–Aug;8(4):230–41.

25 Suzuki S, Komori M, Hirai M, Ureshino N, Kimura S. Development of a novel, fully-automated genotyping system: principle and applications. Sensors. 2012 Dec 3;12(12):16614–27.

26 Suzuki S, Matsusaka S, Hirai M, Shibata H, Takagi K, Mizunuma N, et al. A novel approach to detect KRAS/BRAF mutation for colon cancer: highly sensitive simultaneous detection of mutations and simple pre-treatment without DNA extraction. Int J Oncol. 2015 Jul;47(1):97–105.

27 Roy Chowdhuri S, Hanson J, Cheng J, Rodriguez-Canales J, Fetsch P, Balis U, et al. Semiautomated laser capture microdissection of lung adenocarcinoma cytology samples. Acta Cytol. 2012;56(6):622–31.

Research Article

Acta Cytologica

Acta Cytologica 2021;65:348–353
DOI: 10.1159/000515976

Received: November 10, 2020
Accepted: March 14, 2021
Published online: June 2, 2021

A Preliminary Study of Deep-Learning Algorithm for Analyzing Multiplex Immunofluorescence Biomarkers in Body Fluid Cytology Specimens

Weibo Yu Elizabeth Rao Curtis D. Chin Josephine S. Aguilar-Jakthong Yunfeng Li Christine Chow Shu Yu (Grace) Wang Jianyu Rao

Department of Pathology and Laboratory Medicine, David Geffen School of Medicine, University of California at Los Angeles (UCLA), Los Angeles, CA, USA

Keywords

Deep-learning algorithm · Multiplex immunofluorescence · Biomarkers

Abstract

Introduction: Multiplex biomarker analysis of cytological body fluid specimens is often used to assist cytologists in distiguishing metastatic cancer cells from reactive mesothelial cells. However, evaluating biomarker expression visually may be challenging, especially when the cells of interest are scant. Deep-learning algorithms (DLAs) may be able to assist cytologists in analyzing multiple biomarker expression at the single cell level in the multiplex fluorescence imaging (MFI) setting. This preliminary study was performed to test the feasibility of using DLAs to identify immunofluorescence-stained metastatic adenocarcinoma cells in body fluid cytology samples. ***Methods:*** A DLA was developed to analyze MFI-stained cells in body fluid cytological samples. A total of 41 pleural fluid samples, comprising of 20 positives and 21 negatives, were retrospectively collected. Multiplex immunofluorescence labeling for MOC31, BerEP4, and calretinin, were performed on cell block sections, and results were analyzed by manual analysis (manual MFI) and DLA analysis (MFI-DLA) independently. ***Results:*** All cases with positive original cytological diagnoses showed positive results either by manual MFI or MFI-DLA, but 2 of the 14 (14.3%) original cytologically negative cases had rare cells with positive MOC31 and/or BerEP4 staining in addition to calretinin. Manual MFI analysis and MFI-DLA showed 100% concordance. ***Conclusion:*** MFI combined with DLA provides a potential tool to assist in cytological diagnosis of metastatic malignancy in body fluid samples. Larger studies are warranted to test the clinical validity of the approach.

Introduction

Distinguishing metastatic adenocarcinoma from reactive mesothelial cells in body fluid cytology can be challenging. Diagnoses often require the assistance of immunohistochemical (IHC) staining for a battery of biomarkers, including biomarkers for mesothelial cells and markers for metastatic malignant glandular epithelial cells. Since IHC-based staining is usually performed 1 biomarker at a time and involves multiple cell block sections, it is often difficult to align the staining pattern of

karger@karger.com
www.karger.com/acy

Karger
OPEN ACCESS

Correspondence to:
Curtis D. Chin, cchin8@gmail.com
Josephine S. Aguilar-Jakthong, jajakthong@gmail.com
Jianyu Rao, jrao@mednet.ucla.edu

biomarkers on cells of interest. This is especially problematic in cases with limited cellularity for evaluation.

One potential solution is multiplex fluorescence imaging (MFI) analysis, which allows simultaneous detection of up to 7 targets with quantification capabilities at high resolution on a single cell basis [1, 2]. This approach has been shown to be applicable in a variety of tissue-based settings. However, visual scoring of multiple biomarkers, particularly in a cell block section, can be challenging and time-consuming.

The development of an image-based automatic analytical system that can determine the expression of multiple biomarkers with greater objectivity and reproducibility, and alleviate the burden on pathologists to make challenging and time-consuming assessments, may have significant clinical implications. Deep-learning combined with digital technologies have potential for performing objective, quantitative assessments for biomarker analysis in the single-cell level [3, 4]. These deep-learning approaches use artificial convolutional neural networks, which can be trained directly from primary data without significant pathologist guidance on annotating morphologic or cytologic features. Studies comparing deep-learning based digital image analysis against manual biomarker assessment have been performed in subtyping breast cancer [5], measuring PD-L1 expression in non-small cell lung cancer [6], and scoring tumor infiltrating lymphocytes in tumor areas [7], with deep-learning methods showing superiority or at least non-inferiority to manual scoring with respect to accuracy and reproducibility.

Here, we present the development of a digital image-based deep-learning algorithm (DLA) for analyzing biomarkers in MFI settings (MFI-DLA). In particular, we report the feasibility of performing DLA on cell block sections of pleural fluid samples.

Methods

Sample Collection

We retrospectively and randomly selected 41 out of a total of 864 pleural fluid cytology specimens from archived cell block samples between 2015 and 2018. Of the 41 pleural fluid specimens selected, 20 were malignant and 21 were benign. All samples were collected in the cytology laboratory at University of California, Los Angeles (UCLA). Patient primary histological and cytology diagnosis were recorded for the analysis. Cases with an equivocal cytology diagnosis (atypical or suspicious) were not included in the study. The study was exempt from UCLA's Institutional Review Board assessment as archived cell blocks were used and no patient identifiers were recorded.

Cell Block Preparation

Pleural effusion samples were each centrifuged at 2,500 rpm for 10 min. Supernatant fluid was discarded and the cell pellet transferred to a 1.5-mL centrifugation tube. One drop of warmed agar was added to each pellet and the samples were quickly agitated. Clots formed within 30–60 s and each sample was subsequently placed in a tissue cassette and processed as routine histology samples.

Multiplex IHC Staining of MOC31, BerEP4, and Calretinin

The paraffin slides were stained using the Opal™ Multiplex IHC Kit (Akoya Bioscences), which utilizes a sequence of antibody-antigen binding, fluorescence staining using HRP-conjugated secondary antibody, and heat-mediated removal of the target-binding complex for subsequent targeting of a different antigenic biomarker. In addition to the greater degree of multiplexing, this kit allows for compatibility with unlabeled primary antibodies, reduced cross-reactivity between antibodies, and no limitations with species compatibility by virtue of serial biomarker staining.

Briefly, cell block sections were dewaxed with xylene, rehydrated with a series of ethanol solutions, and washed. Antigen retrieval was performed using microwave treatment (45 s at 100% power, then additional 15 min at 20% power) with AR buffer (AR6 or AR9, Akoya Bioscences), then the slides were blocked, cooled, and washed with distilled water and TBST. Slides were incubated with primary antibodies specific to calretinin (Invitrogen, Cat#:180211, 1:100 dilution), Moc31 (Dako, #M3525, 1:200 dilution), and BerEP4 (Dako, #M0804, 1:200 dilution). Slides were then incubated with secondary anti-rabbit HRP-conjugated antibody (Dako envision, #K4003) or anti-mouse HRP-conjugated antibody (Dako envision, #K4001). Then a signal amplification of Opal fluorophore (1:100 dilution at room temperature for 10 min), followed by additional microwave treatment (45 s at 100% power, then additional 15 min at 20% power) between each antibody staining, and a final application of DAPI counterstain (1:2,000 dilution for 5 min) was performed. The fluorophores used were Opal 520 FITC for calretinin; Opal 570 TRITC for Moc31; and Opal 650 CY5 for BerE4. Fluorescence image exposure times are as follows: DAPI: 3.977 ms, FITC (OPAL 520): calretinin 37.27 ms, Cy3 (OPAL 570): MOC31 35.856 ms, and Cy5 (OPAL 690): BerEP4 39.09 ms. The images were then scanned at ×20 magnification (Vectra Polaris, Akoya) and uploaded to a secure UCLA file share system.

Visiopharm APP Development for Analyzing Biomarkers in Multiplex Settings

We designed the multiplexed biomarker analysis protocol package (APP) with Visiopharm, a company that specializes in developing image analysis software using DLA (https://www.visiopharm.com). The APP was designed to allow biomarker combinations to be analyzed, provided that the panels (1) used DAPI nuclei stain to highlight nucleated cells, (2) included a total of 4 stains, (3) used identical fluorophores (FITC, TRITC, CY5, and DAPI), and (4) scanned each fluorophore channel in the order performed for images on the training dataset. In addition, while the APP was initially validated on whole ovarian tumor tissue slides cut from formalin-fixed paraffin embedded tissue blocks, the APP has the capability of evaluating multiplexed biomarker expression on cytology specimen preparations such as aspirate smears, cytospins, and cell blocks, so long as the above criteria are met. The APP was also partitioned into several "sub-protocols,"

Acta Cytologica 2021;65:348–353
DOI: 10.1159/000515976

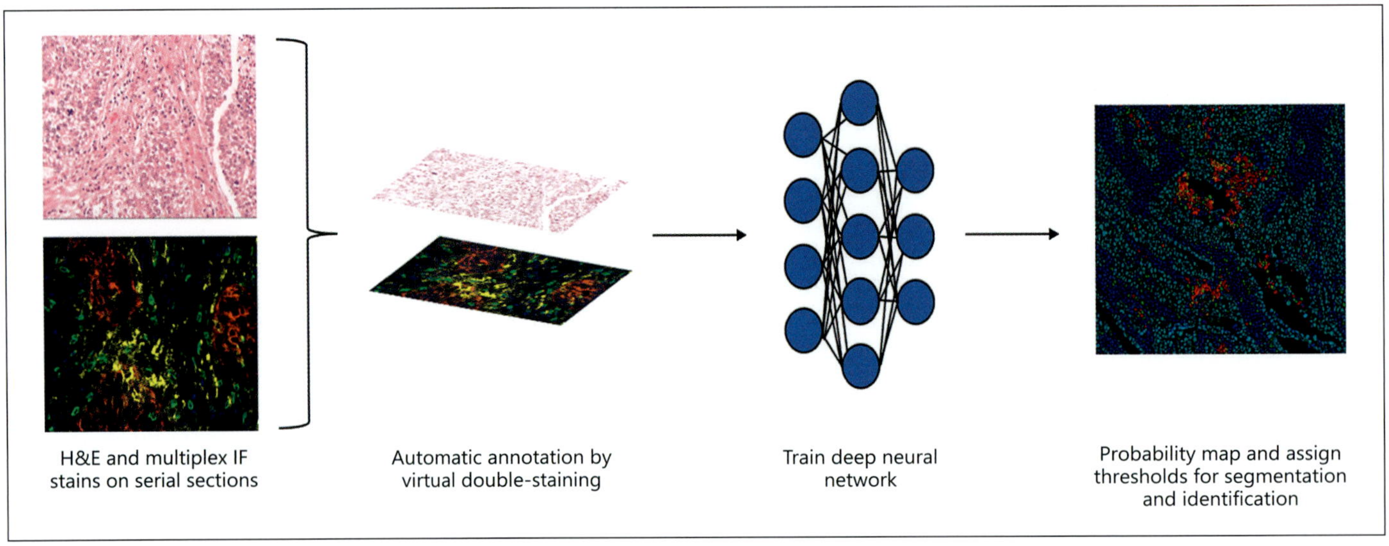

Fig. 1. Schematic of overall process for developing DLA for MFI analysis on sections. DLA, deep-learning algorithm; MFI, multiplex fluorescence imaging.

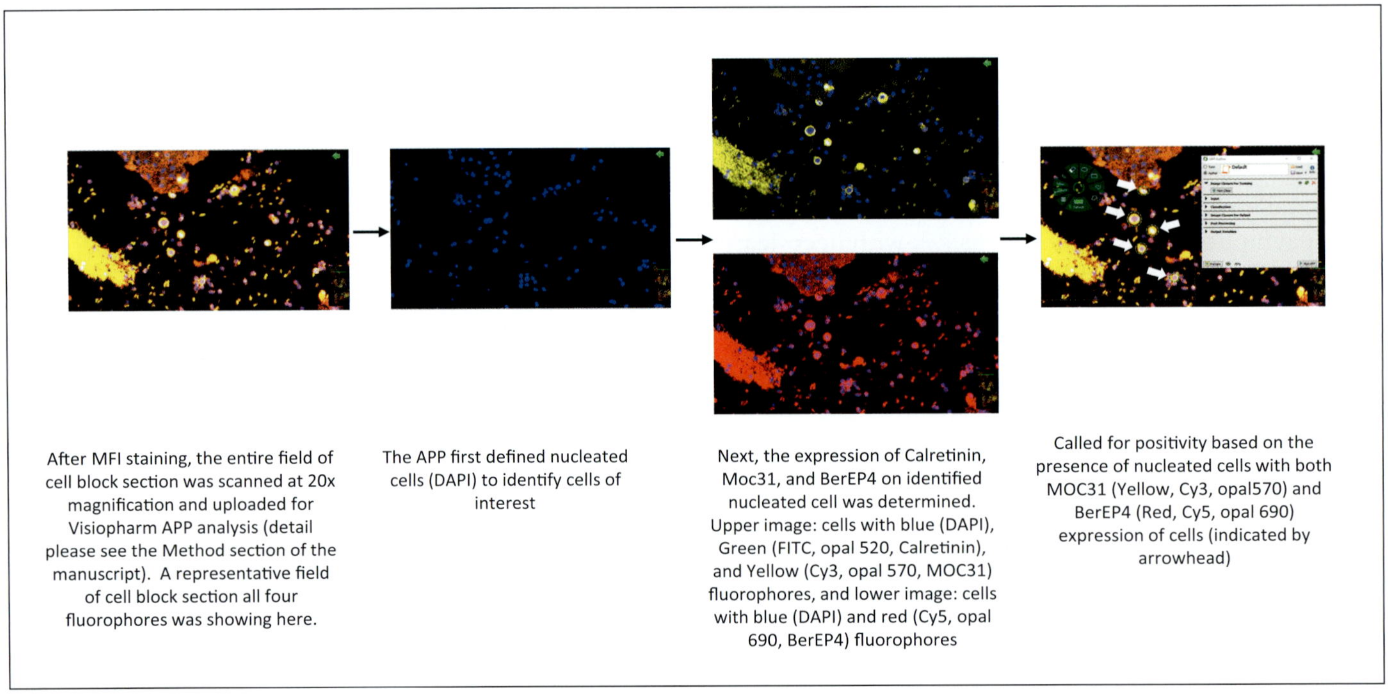

Fig. 2. The process of how positivity for metastatic tumor cells based on MOC31 and BerEP4 was determined by DLA (Visiopharm APP) with an example of a positive case of the study. All images shown were taken at 20× magnification.

namely tumor/stroma segmentation (not used in the cell block setting), cell identification, and DAPI quantification on a region of interest (for detecting aneuploidy or polyploidy). This separation was implemented to allow the end-user to select functions based on the clinical situation and avoid wasting time on computational tasks that were not needed.

A significant challenge in developing DLA is curating a high-quality training dataset. Traditionally, this training dataset re-

Table 1. Primary cytology diagnosis and the results of MFI visual analysis and MFI-DLA analysis

	Cytology diagnosis	MFI biomarker staining		MFI results	MFI-DLA results
		calretinin	MOC31/BerEP4		
1	Adenocarcinoma	Negative	Positive	Positive	Positive
2	Adenocarcinoma	Negative	Positive	Positive	Positive
3	Adenocarcinoma	Negative	Positive	Positive	Positive
4	Adenocarcinoma	Negative	Positive	Positive	Positive
5	Adenocarcinoma	Positive	Positive	Positive	Positive
6	Adenocarcinoma	Negative	Positive	Positive	Positive
7	Adenocarcinoma	Positive	Positive	Positive	Positive
8	Adenocarcinoma	Positive	Positive	Positive	Positive
9	Adenocarcinoma	Positive	Positive	Positive	Positive
10	Adenocarcinoma	Positive	Positive	Positive	Positive
11	Adenocarcinoma	Positive	Positive	Positive	Positive
12	Adenocarcinoma	Positive	Positive	Positive	Positive
13	Adenocarcinoma	Positive	Positive	Positive	Positive
14	Adenocarcinoma	Positive	Positive	Positive	Positive
15	Adenocarcinoma	Negative	Positive	Positive	Positive
16	Adenocarcinoma	Negative	Positive	Positive	Positive
17	Adenocarcinoma	Positive	Positive	Positive	Positive
18	Supportive of carcinoma	Positive	Positive	Positive	Positive
19	Adenocarcinoma	Positive	Positive	Positive	Positive
20	Adenocarcinoma	Positive	Positive	Positive	Positive
21	Negative	Positive	Negative	Negative	Negative
22	Reactive changes	Positive	Negative	Negative	Negative
23	Negative	Positive	Negative	Negative	Negative
24	Negative	Positive	Negative	Negative	Negative
25	Negative	Positive	Negative	Negative	Negative
26	Reactive changes	Positive	Negative	Negative	Negative
27	Negative	Positive	Negative	Negative	Negative
28	Negative	Positive	Negative	Negative	Negative
29	Negative	Positive	Negative	Negative	Negative
30	Negative	Positive	Negative	Negative	Negative
31	Negative	Positive	Negative	Negative	Negative
32	Negative	Positive	Negative	Negative	Negative
33	Negative	Positive	Positive	Equivocal	Equivocal
34	Negative	Positive	Positive	Equivocal	Equivocal

DLA, deep-learning algorithm; MFI, multiplex fluorescence imaging.

quires a pathologist to manually annotate enough features (roughly 1,000 objects), which is very time-consuming. To solve this challenge, our APP used automatic annotation by a process known as virtual double-staining, which aligns serial H&E and MFI sections so that information on the MFI can be transferred to H&E without manually annotating the H&E. These automatic annotations are then fed into a deep neural network; once trained, the APP can receive a new sample, create a probability map of likely areas of biomarker expression or features of interest, and assign a probability threshold percentage to then perform segmentation or identification (Fig. 1). The end result is a faster, more precise, and scalable curation of training data.

Interpretation of Results and Statistical Analysis

Manual MFI and MFI-DLA used the same criteria to determine if the specimen was "positive" or "negative" for metastatic malignancy: if there were cells which stained positive for MOC31 and/or BerEP4 and negative for calretinin, then the specimen was scored positive. Otherwise, the specimen was considered negative. Cells which stained positive for calretinin (green fluorescence) with additional MOC31 (yellow fluorescence) and/or BerEP4 (red fluorescence) positivity were considered equivocal. MFI analysis was carried out 6 months after manual MFI analysis as a washout period. Diagnoses from visual scoring and DLA scoring were compared with patient's primary diagnosis and cytology diagnosis. Final results were confirmed by 2 pathologists (J.A.J. and J.Y.R.).

Results and Discussion

A total of 41 cases of pleural fluids, of which 20 were malignant and 21 were benign, were selected for the study. Seven of the 21 benign cases were noted to have only red blood cells on the cell blocks. These cases were excluded, leaving a total of 14 benign cases. The analysis process and staining patterns of MOC31, BerEP4 and calretinin are shown in Figure 2. DLA scoring generated the same results as the visual scoring (100% concordance, Table 1). While all cases with positive original cytological diagnoses showed positive visual MFI and MFI-DLA scores, 2 of the 14 (14.3%) original cytologically negative cases had rare calretinin positive cells that also stained positive for MOC31 and/or BerEP4. These 2 cases were considered "equivocal" by MFI and MFI-DLA analysis.

While initially validated on histological sections, the APP was designed with enough flexibility for analyzing cytology specimens with different cell markers expressed on heterogeneous cell populations. Here, we reported the results of DLA scoring for analyzing biomarkers in a multiplex immunofluorescence setting. Although only 34 cases were included in final analysis, our study demonstrated the feasibility of MFI-DLA analysis with complete (100%) concordance with manual MFI analysis.

It is interesting that 2 of the original cytologically negative cases had rare cells with MOC31 and/or BerEP4 positivity. This is not surprising as neither MOC31 nor BerEP4 antibody are 100% specific for identifying metastatic adenocarcinoma. MOC31 and BerEP4 expression may be seen in cases of reactive mesothelial cells at frequencies up to 13 and 10%, respectively [8, 9]. Albeit there were occasional nonspecific expressions of MOC31 or BerEP4 in mesothelial cells, a significant finding of 100% concordance between the manual score and DLA score was noted. These findings highlight the potential application of MFI-DLA in determining metastatic malignancies in body fluid cytological specimens.

Another interesting finding was the variable cellularity across the entire dataset; Figure 2 shows a typical positive case. In this study, the percentage of positive tumor cells in relation to mesothelial cells was not measured as it did not affect/contribute the outcome (positive or negative for tumor cells), though we acknowledge that this would be interesting to characterize in a future study.

While the preliminary study demonstrated the potential application of our MFI-DLA in differentiating metastatic malignancy versus benign pleural fluid samples, this approach may be useful in other settings important for diagnosis and management of cancer, such as quantifying PD-L1, Her-2, P16, and Ki-67 expression in single-cell levels. In fact, the program was developed initially for the analysis of PD-L1 in MFI setting. However, carefully designed studies will be needed to validate the value of MFI-DLA in actual clinical settings.

In conclusion, it is feasible to perform MFI-DLA analysis on cell block sections from body fluid samples. While most DLA methods have been validated on histology specimens, there may also be value in applying these tools to cytology specimens in clinical settings where fluids and cellular aspirates are more accessible and convenient to obtain. However, the actual clinical utility of this approach remains to be determined in additional studies with larger sample sizes.

Acknowledgements

We thank Sarah Holm Jørgensen from Visiopharm for technical expertise and support in APP development.

Statement of Ethics

The project received exemption from Institutional Review Board for human research subjects at UCLA.

Conflict of Interest Statement

The authors have no conflicts of interest to declare.

Funding Sources

Project funded internally by the research fund of Department of Pathology and Laboratory Medicine, UCLA.

Author Contributions

Jianyu Rao conceptualized the study. Curtis Chin worked with Visiopharm to develop MFI-DLA program, Josephine S. Aguilar-Jakthong and Yunfeng Li prepared the cases and performed the stains and manual analysis. Weibo Yu performed MFI-DLA analysis. Elizabeth Rao, Christine Chow, and Grace Wang were student volunteers in Jianyu Rao's group who worked with Weibo Yu virtually to carry out MFI-DLA analysis and manuscript preparation.

References

1 Viratham Pulsawatdi A, Craig SG, Bingham V, McCombe K, Humphries MP, Senevirathne S, et al. A robust multiplex immunofluorescence and digital pathology workflow for the characterisation of the tumour immune microenvironment. Mol Oncol. 2020 Oct;14(10):2384–402.

2 Tan WCC, Nerurkar SN, Cai HY, Ng HHM, Wu D, Wee YTF, et al. Overview of multiplex immunohistochemistry/immunofluorescence techniques in the era of cancer immunotherapy. Cancer Commun. 2020;40(4):135–53.

3 Bera K, Schalper KA, Rimm DL, Velcheti V, Madabhushi A. Artificial intelligence in digital pathology: new tools for diagnosis and precision oncology. Nat Rev Clin Oncol. 2019;16(11):703–15.

4 Niazi MKK, Parwani AV, Gurcan MN. Digital pathology and artificial intelligence. Lancet Oncol. 2019;20(5):e253–61.

5 Stalhammar G, Fuentes Martinez N, Lippert M, Tobin NP, Mølholm I, Kis L, et al. Digital image analysis outperforms manual biomarker assessment in breast cancer. Mod Pathol. 2016;29(4):318–29.

6 Kapil A, Meier A, Zuraw A, Steele KE, Rebelatto MC, Schmidt G, et al. Deep semi supervised generative learning for automated tumor proportion scoring on NSCLC tissue needle biopsies. Sci Rep. 2018;8(1):17343.

7 Klauschen F, Müller KR, Binder A, Bockmayr M, Hägele M, Seegerer P, et al. Scoring of tumor-infiltrating lymphocytes: from visual estimation to deep learning. Semin Cancer Biol. 2018;52(Pt 2):151–7.

8 Arora R, Agarwal S, Mathur SR, Verma K, Iyer VK, Aron M. Utility of a limited panel of calretinin and Ber-EP4 immunocytochemistry on cytospin preparation of serous effusions: a cost-effective measure in resource-limited settings. Cytojournal. 2011;8:14.

9 Kundu UR, Krishnamurthy S. Use of the monoclonal antibody MOC-31 as an immunomarker for detecting metastatic adenocarcinoma in effusion cytology. Cancer Cytopathol. 2011;119(4):272–8.

Commentary

Acta Cytologica

Acta Cytologica 2021;65:354–357
DOI: 10.1159/000518382

Received: May 31, 2021
Accepted: July 7, 2021
Published online: July 20, 2021

A Machine Learning Tool Using Digital Microscopy (Morphogo) for the Identification of Abnormal Lymphocytes in the Bone Marrow

Gusheng Tang[a] Xinyan Fu[b] Zhen Wang[c] Mingyi Chen[d]

[a]Department of Hematology, Changhai Hospital, Shanghai, China; [b]Division of Medical Technology Development, Hangzhou ZhiWei Information and Technology Co. Ltd., Hangzhou, China; [c]Clinical Laboratory, The First Affiliated Hospital of Dalian Medical University, Dalian, China; [d]Department of Pathology and Laboratory Medicine, University of Texas, Southwestern Medical Center, Dallas, TX, USA

Keywords

Digital pathology · Machine learning · Morphological analysis · Bone marrow · Lymphocyte

Abstract

Morphological analysis of the bone marrow is an essential step in the diagnosis of hematological disease. The conventional analysis of bone marrow smears is performed under a manual microscope, which is labor-intensive and subject to interobserver variability. The morphological differential diagnosis of abnormal lymphocytes from normal lymphocytes is still challenging. The digital pathology methods integrated with advances in machine learning enable new diagnostic features/algorithms from digital bone marrow cell images in order to optimize classification, thus providing a robust and faster screening diagnostic tool. We have developed a machine learning system, Morphogo, based on algorithms to discriminate abnormal lymphocytes from normal lymphocytes using digital imaging analysis. We retrospectively reviewed 347 cases of bone marrow digital images. Among them, 53 cases had a clinical history and the diagnosis of marrow involvement with lymphoma was confirmed either by morphology or flow cytometry. We split the 53 cases into two groups for training and testing with 43 and 10 cases, respectively. The selected 15,353 cell images were reviewed by pathologists, based on morphological visual appearance, from 43 patients whose diagnosis was confirmed by complementary tests. To expand the range and the precision of recognizing the lymphoid cells in the marrow by automated digital microscopy systems, we developed an algorithm that incorporated color and texture in addition to geometrical cytological features of the variable lymphocyte images which were applied as the training data set. The selected images from the 10 patients were analyzed by the trained artificial intelligence-based recognition system and compared with the final diagnosis rendered by pathologists. The positive predictive value for the identification of the categories of reactive/normal lymphocytes and abnormal lymphoid cells was 99.04%. It seems likely that further training and improvement of the algorithms will facilitate further subclassification of specific lineage subset pathology, e.g., diffuse large B-cell lymphoma from chronic lymphocytic leukemia/small lymphocytic lymphoma, follicular lymphoma, mantle cell lymphoma or even hairy cell leukemia in cases of abnormal malignant lymphocyte classes in the future. This research demonstrated the feasibility of digital pathology and emerging machine learning approaches to automatically diagnose lymphoma cells in the bone marrow based on cytological-histological analyses.

Correspondence to:
Mingyi Chen, mingyi.chen@utsouthwestern.edu

Introduction

Despite the impressive advances in molecular pathology, morphological analysis of bone marrow smears remains the fundamental step to identify the various subtypes of cells in the initial diagnosis of hematological diseases. Traditionally, the counting and classification of the bone marrow cells relies on manual differential count under light microscopy by pathologists and other well-trained laboratory personnel. This time-consuming diagnostic procedure is subjective and dependent on the practitioner's experience. Furthermore, the variability of criteria and potential selection bias of cells in the slides may yield intra- and interobserver variances.

The emerging technologies integrating high-resolution digital pathology and machine learning tools reformed the tedious manual process with a highly efficient automated platform in diagnostic hematology [1]. Therefore, the computer-assisted diagnosis system for bone marrow differentiation is pursued for practical applications. In the last decade, the most successful progress in automated analysis was the application in peripheral blood smears, followed by breakthroughs in bone marrow smears and histopathology (bone marrow biopsies) [1].

A representative digital morphology microscopy system is "Morphogo" [2], which allows batch automated analysis of bone marrow smears, scanning the smear (20 mm × 40 mm) and generating a whole slide image (0.17 ± 0.02 μm/pixel) of the bone marrow smear, then automatically acquire, segment and identify nucleated cells in the digital image at a magnification of ×1,000 (×100 oil, 0.018 ± 0.005 μm/pixel) [3], finally generate an auxiliary report of the bone marrow smear. The system has established a digital analysis process required for the morphological analysis of bone marrow smears. It is expected to improve the efficiency and accuracy in the diagnosis of hematological diseases. The findings were initially presented at the USCAP meeting in March 2019. Recently, the validation study has been published. It demonstrated a recognition rate of 85.7% of nucleated cells in bone marrow and a high agreement between the percentage of cell series by the automatic system and those by manual count under the light microscope [2]. This system is still in the early phase of clinical diagnostic implementation and is currently more used for telepathology consultation and research projects. It is proved to be a useful screening tool to discriminate abnormal nucleated cells from normal hematopoietic cells, it has the potential to optimize the work flow of pathologists in the daily practice of hematopathology. Plasma cells and mature lymphocytes also displayed a good correlation [2].

Digital Morphology Analysis of Lymphoma Cells in Bone Marrow Smears

A careful multiparametric approach in bone marrow study plays a pivotal role for the initial investigation of specimens of lymphoma as well as staging lymphoma. The identification of abnormal lymphocytes in the bone marrow is the initial step in the diagnosis of malignant lymphoma or clinical staging.

We integrate high-resolution digital images and a machine learning approach of new diagnostic features/algorithms to optimize the process of classification of marrow cells, thus providing a robust and faster screening diagnostic tool. Early studies confirmed the feasibility of automatic screening and identification of reactive and abnormal lymphocytes in the peripheral blood smear [4], as well as whole slide imaging-based primary diagnosis of lymphoma using marrow biopsy samples [5]. Therefore, it is appealing to develop a computer-aided automatic analysis system on bone marrow smears in order to aid diagnosis and interpretation of potential lymphoma involvement.

The Morphogo system was validated to recognize lymphocytes in the differential from other lineages of bone marrow hematopoietic cells; the results have already been published in our previous studies [2]. The accuracy of recognition of lymphocytes in bone marrow aspirate smears by the instrument was 87.8% (sensitivity 85.5% and specificity 88.3%). In this current review article, we focused on the ongoing progress of automatic recognition of large atypical lymphocytes. Recently, we have trained the Morphogo system to identify abnormal lymphocytes in marrow smears using digital imaging analysis. The result was presented in the most recent ISLH meeting in May 2021. We retrospectively reviewed 347 cases of staging bone marrow smears with a clinical history of lymphomas. Among them, 53 cases had bone marrow involvement with lymphomas confirmed by morphology and/or flow cytometry. We split the 53 cases into two groups, 43 cases for training and 10 cases for further testing (Table 1). The selected 15,353 high-resolution images of lymphocytes reviewed by pathologists were used as training data sets. To expand the range and the precision of recognizing the lymphoid cells in the bone marrow by the system, we developed an algorithm that incorporated cell size, nuclear/cytoplasmic color and texture in

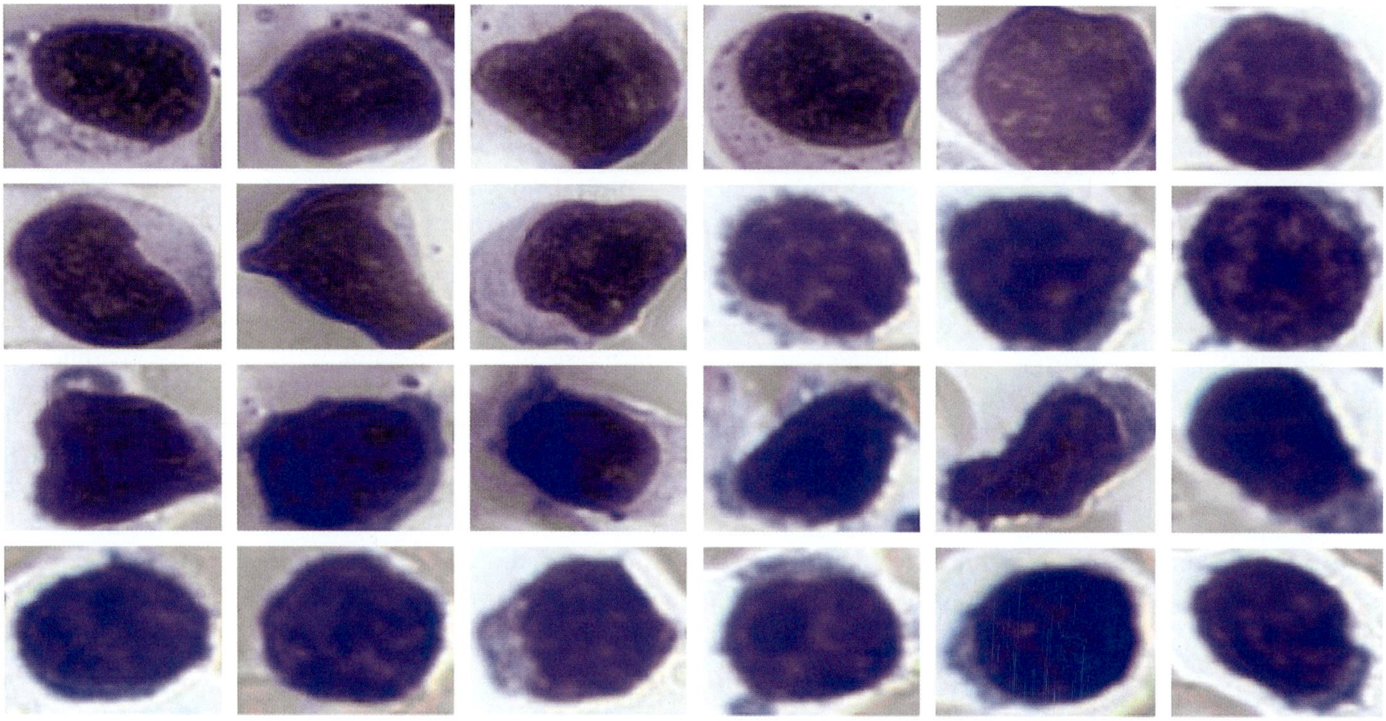

Fig. 1. Selected representative digital images of abnormal large atypical lymphocytes from cases of large B-cell lymphoma or high-grade follicular lymphoma.

Table 1. Summary of the cases of bone marrow with diagnosis of lymphomas

Diagnosis	Training				Diagnosis	Testing			
	cases	images	audit cells	acquired cells		cases	images	audit cells	acquired cells
BLL	1	486	10	21	BLL	1	465	54	58
CLL	2	743	530	473	DLBCL	3	927	198	202
DLBCL	18	6,676	1,434	1,501	MZL	1	299	35	35
FL	1	372	77	102	NHL	5	1,925	538	538
Unclassified Lymphoma	2	541	134	137	Total	10	3,616	825	833
MCL	1	359	62	63					
NHL	16	5,579	1,859	1,939					
TLL	2	597	326	343					
Total	43	15,353	4,432	4,579					

BLL, B-lymphoblastic lymphoma; TLL, T-lymphoblastic lymphoma; CLL, chronic lymphocytic leukemia; DLBCL, diffuse large B-cell lymphoma; FL, follicular lymphoma; MCL, mantle cell lymphoma; MZL, marginal zone lymphoma; NHL, non-Hodgkin lymphoma.

addition to geometrical cytological features of the variable lymphocyte images, which were used as the training data set. The selected images from the 10 patients with large B-cell lymphoma or high-grade follicular lymphoma were analyzed by the trained artificial intelligence-based recognition system and compared with the final diagnosis rendered by pathologists (Fig. 1). The positive predictive value for the identification of the categories of abnormal lymphoid cells was 99.04%. Due to the subtle morphological changes, the attempts to discriminate small lymphocytes from the spectrum of maturation stages of hematogones are still challenging [6]. As a screening tool, the Morphogo system is reliable in the identification of a higher percentage of lymphocyte count (>20%) or lower-level large atypical lymphocytes (>5%) [2]. There are still some limitations in the quantification of lymphocytes in the marrow smears due to the sampling discrepancy and paratrabecular lymphoid aggregates in the marrow core biopsy. Therefore, the Morphogo system is a useful ancillary tool, but not for the final diagnosis; the final interpretation always needs to be correlated with the findings of bone marrow core biopsy, flow cytometry and molecular study results.

Combining digital pathology methods with advanced machine learning, developing new digital cell image diagnostic features/algorithms, continuously optimizing cell classification and incorporating diagnostic screening into the pathology workflow will help pathologists in the diagnosis of malignant lymphoma [6]. In spite of the technological challenges, we are optimistic about the progress of ongoing research based on a large data set of lymphoma cases from a multicenter study for further training and testing; the success will help to deploy it into real-world clinical practice of digital hematopathology.

Suggestions for Improvement

It is expected that further training and improvement of the mathematic algorithms will facilitate the detection and further subclassification of abnormal lymphocytes, e.g., diffuse large B-cell lymphoma from chronic lymphocytic leukemia/small lymphocytic lymphoma, low-grade follicular lymphoma or conventional mantle cell lymphoma, in the near future [6].

Conclusion

Bone marrow study including aspiration and biopsy is regarded as the standard for staging lymphoma patients. Advances in digital pathology and artificial intelligence have allowed a digital process of morphological analysis of bone marrow for the early diagnosis or staging of hematological disorders such as lymphoma and myeloma. This preliminary data demonstrated the feasibility of digital pathology coupled with emerging machine learning approaches to automatically identify abnormal lymphocytes in the bone marrow and diagnose lymphoma based on cytological-histological analyses.

Acknowledgement

The authors would like to acknowledge Dr. Chuhu Yang for guidance and proofreading of the article.

Conflict of Interest Statement

Xinyan Fu is an employee of Hangzhou ZhiWei Information & Technology Co. Ltd. Mingyi Chen is in the advisory board and received research grant support from A lab/ZhiWei Information & Technology Co. Ltd. The other authors have no conflicts of interest to declare.

Funding Sources

This work was supported by Hangzhou ZhiWei Information & Technology Co. Ltd.

Author Contributions

Writing – original draft preparation, review and editing: Gusheng Tang, Xinyan Fu, Zhen Wang and Mingyi Chen. All authors have read and agreed to the final paper for submission.

References

1 Radakovich N, Nagy M, Nazha A. Machine learning in haematological malignancies. Lancet Haematol. 2020 Jul;7(7):e541–50.
2 Fu X, Fu M, Li Q, Peng X, Lu J, Fang F, et al. Morphogo: an automatic bone marrow cell classification system on digital images analyzed by artificial intelligence. Acta Cytol. 2020;64(6):588–96.
3 Jin H, Fu X, Cao X, Sun M, Wang X, Zhong Y, et al. Developing and preliminary validating an automatic cell classification system for bone marrow smears: a pilot study. J Med Syst. 2020 Sep;44(10):184.
4 Alférez S, Merino A, Bigorra L, Mujica L, Ruiz M, Rodellar J. Automatic recognition of atypical lymphoid cells from peripheral blood by digital image analysis. Am J Clin Pathol. 2015 Feb;143(2):168–76.
5 Miyoshi H, Sato K, Kabeya Y, Yonezawa S, Nakano H, Takeuchi Y, et al. Deep learning shows the capability of high-level computer-aided diagnosis in malignant lymphoma. Lab Invest. 2020 Oct;100(10):1300–10.
6 Alférez S, Merino A, Mujica LE, Ruiz M, Bigorra L, Rodellar J. Automatic classification of atypical lymphoid B cells using digital blood image processing. Int J Lab Hematol. 2014 Aug;36(4):472–80.

Acta Cytologica

Author Index Vol. 65, No. 4, 2021

Subject Index Vol. 65, No. 4, 2021

karger@karger.com
www.karger.com/acy

Karger

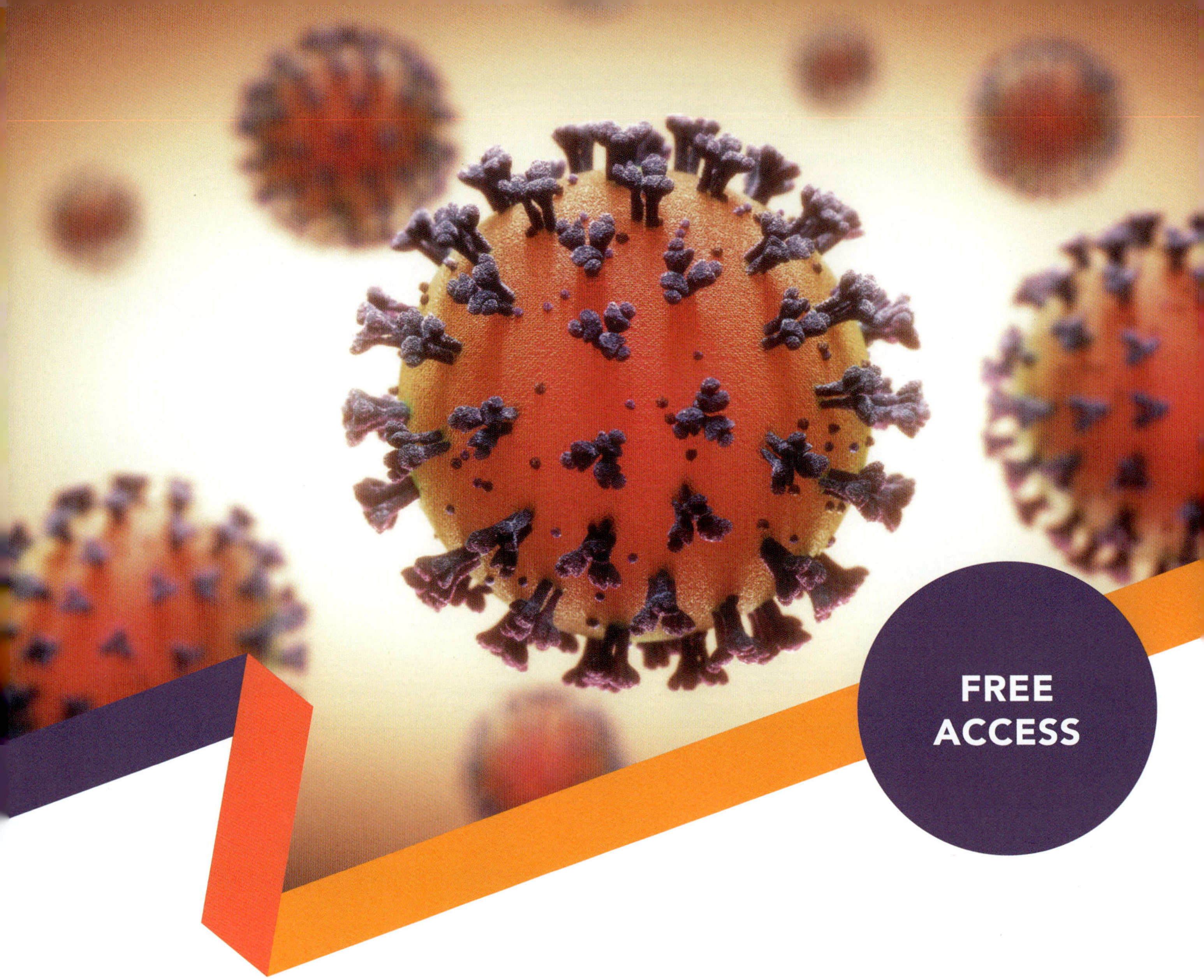
FREE
ACCESS